Lecture Notes of the Institute for Computer Sciences, Social Informatics and Telecommunications Engineering   187

More information about this series at http://www.springer.com/series/8197

Mobyen Uddin Ahmed · Shahina Begum
Wasim Raad (Eds.)

Internet of Things Technologies for HealthCare

Third International Conference, HealthyIoT 2016
Västerås, Sweden, October 18–19, 2016
Revised Selected Papers

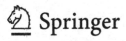 Springer

Editors
Mobyen Uddin Ahmed
School Innovation, Design, Engineering
Märlardalen University
Västerås
Sweden

Shahina Begum
School Innovation, Design, Engineering
Mälardalen University
Västerås
Sweden

Wasim Raad
Computer Engineering Department
King Fahd University of Petroleum and
   Minerals
Dhahran
Saudi Arabia

ISSN 1867-8211   ISSN 1867-822X   (electronic)
Lecture Notes of the Institute for Computer Sciences, Social Informatics
and Telecommunications Engineering
ISBN 978-3-319-51233-4   ISBN 978-3-319-51234-1   (eBook)
DOI 10.1007/978-3-319-51234-1

Library of Congress Control Number: 2016960780

Printed on acid-free paper

This Springer imprint is published by Springer Nature
The registered company is Springer International Publishing AG
The registered company address is: Gewerbestrasse 11, 6330 Cham, Switzerland

Preface

The EAI International Conference on IoT Technologies for HealthCare (HealthyIoT) focuses on Internet of Things (IoT) technologies for health care. The 2016 conference was the third scientific event in the series bringing together expertise from technological, medical, social, and political domains. The IoT, as a set of existing and emerging technologies, notions, and services, can provide many solutions for the delivery of electronic health care, patient care, and medical data management. The event brought together technology experts, researchers, industry and international authorities contributing toward the assessment, development, and deployment of health care solutions based on IoT technologies, standards, and procedures. HealthyIoT 2016 also included the First Workshop on Emerging eHealth through Internet of Things (EHIoT 2016). Thus, it opened a new chapter in the success story of the series of international conferences on HealthyIoT by presenting keynotes, oral presentations, short poster presentations, and the workshop provided by more than 100 authors from 15 countries from various parts of the world.

HealthyIoT 2016 benefited from the experience and the lessons learned from the Organizing Committees of previous HealthyIoT events, particularly HealthyIoT 2014 and HealthyIoT 2015. Both conferences were co-located events that took place in Rome, Italy, forming one of the main conferences of the IoT360 Summit. The conferences were organized by CREATE-NET in collaboration with the European Alliance for Innovation in Slovakia, and its partner, the European Alliance for Innovation in Trento, Italy. Additionaly, HealthyIoT 2015 also included the First Workshop on Embedded Sensor Systems for Health through Internet of Things (ESS-H IoT 2015) with the aim of using embedded sensor systems in health monitoring applications considering the future vision of IoT.

This proceedings volume comprises a total of 31 research papers out of 43 submissions, with contributions by researchers across Europe and around the world. Among them, 20 oral presentations to the HealthyIoT 2016 conference, eight poster presentations, and three oral presentations to the EHIoT 2016 workshop. All submissions were carefully and critically reviewed by at least two independent experts from the scientific Program Committee and international reviewers. The highly selective review process resulted in an acceptance rate of 72%, thereby guaranteeing a high scientific level of the accepted and finally published papers. The publication includes manuscripts written and presented by authors from different countries, including the UK, Sweden, Turkey, Japan, Belgium, Saudi Arabia, United States, Portugal, Italy, Thailand, Slovakia, France, Pakistan, Australia, and Bosnia and Herzegovina. Topics including "Health-Care Support for the Elderly," "Real-Time Monitoring Systems," "Security, Safety and Communication," "Smart Homes and Smart Caring Environments," "Intelligent Data Processing and Predictive Algorithms in eHealth," "Emerging eHealth IoT Applications," "Signal Processing and Analysis," and "The Smartphone as a HealthyThing," are covered.

The HealthyIoT 2016 conference would not have been possible without the supporters and sponsors including the European Alliance for Innovation (EAI), CREATE-NET, Springer, Mälardalen University, Microsoft, and other the local sponsors.

The editors are also grateful to the dedicated efforts of the Organizing Committee members and their supporters for carefully and smoothly preparing and operating the conference. They especially thank all team members from the Embedded Sensor Systems for Health, Mälardalen University, Västerås, Sweden, for their dedication to the event. In conclusion, we would like to once again express our sincere thanks to all the authors and attendees of the conference in Västerås, Sweden, and also the authors who contributed to the creation of this HealhthyIoT 2016 publication.

November 2016   Mobyen Uddin Ahmed
                                                 Shahina Begum
                                                 Wasim Raad

Organization

The 3rd EAI International Conference on IoT Technologies for HealthCare

General Chair

Mobyen Uddin Ahmed   Mälardalen University, Sweden

Steering Committee Chair

Imrich Chlamtac   President of Create-Net, President of European Alliance for Innovation, Italy

Steering Committee

Joel J.P.C. Rodrigues	Instituto de Telecomunicações, University of Beira Interior, Portugal
Antonio J. Jara	Institute of Information Systems, University of Applied Sciences Western Switzerland (HES-SO), Switzerland
Shoumen Palit Austin Datta	School of Engineering Massachusetts Institute of Technology; Industrial Internet Consortium, USA
Arijit Ukil	Tata Consultancy Services, India

Technical Program Chairs

Antonio J. Jara	Institute of Information Systems, University of Applied Sciences Western Switzerland (HES-SO), Switzerland
Stefania Montani	DISIT - Computer Science Institute, Italy
Shahina Begum	Mälardalen University, Sweden
Diego Gachet Páez	Universidad Europea de Madrid, Spain

Publications Chairs

Wasim Raad	King Fahd University of Petroleum and Minerals, Saudi Arabia
Shahina Begum	Mälardalen University, Sweden

Program Committee

Jesus Favela	CICESE, Mexico
Marcela Rodriguez	UABC, Mexico
Manuel de Buenaga	Universidad Europea de Madrid, Spain
Carmelo R. García	Universidad de Las Palmas de Gran Canaria, Spain
Ramiro Delgado	Army Forces University, Ecuador
Kunal Mankodiya	University of Rhode Island, USA
Malcolm Clarke	Brunel University, UK
Emilija Stojmenova Duh	University of Ljubljana, Slovenia
Yunchuan Sun	China University of Geosciences (Beijing), China
Enrique Puertas	Universidad Europea de Madrid, Spain
Alan Jovic	University of Zagreb, Croatia
Ahsan Khandoker	Khalifa University, United Arab Emirates
Mobyen Uddin Ahmed	Mälardalen University, Sweden
Venet Osmani	CREATE-NET, Italy
Faisal Shaikh	Mehran University of Engineering and Technology, Pakistan
Emad Felemban	Science and Technology Unit, UQU University, Makkah, Saudi Arabia
Silvia Gabrielli	CREATE-NET, Italy
Gregory Abowd	Gatech, USA
Arijit Ukil	Scientist R&D, Tata Consultancy Services, India
Mosabber Uddin Ahmed	University of Dhaka, Bangladesh
Rossi Kamal	Kyung Hee University, South Korea
Stefano Tennina	University of L'Aquila, Italy
Mário Alves	Polytechnic Institute of Porto (ISEP/IPP), Portugal
Anis Koubâa	Prince Sultan University, Saudi Arabia
Ramiro Martinez de Dios	University of Seville, Spain
Shashi Prabh	Shiv Nadar University, India
Carlo Alberto Boano	TU Graz, Austria
Behnam Dezfouli	University of Iowa, USA

Sponsorship and Exhibit Chairs

Kristina Lukacova	European Alliance for Innovation, Slovakia
Therese Jagestig Bjurquist	Mälardalen University, Sweden

Workshops Chair

Aida Čaušević	Mälardalen University, Sweden

Publicity and Social Media Chair

Hossein Fotouhi	Mälardalen University, Sweden

Web Chair

Shaibal Barua   Mälardalen University, Sweden

Local Chairs

Hossein Fotouhi   Mälardalen University, Sweden
Aida Čaušević   Mälardalen University, Sweden

Advisors

Maria Lindén   Mälardalen University, Sweden
Mats Björkman   Mälardalen University, Sweden

Conference Manager

Lenka Laukova   EAI - European Alliance for Innovation

Workshop on Emerging eHealth through Internet of Things

Organizing Committee

Almir Badnjević   International Burch University and University of
                           Sarajevo, Bosnia and Herzegovina
Radovan Stojanović   University of Montenegro, Montenegro
Mario Cifrek   University of Zagreb, Croatia

Program Committee

Thomas Penzel   Charite University Hospital Berlin, Germany
Leonardo Bocchi   University of Florence, Italy
Damir Marjanović   International Burch University, Bosnia and
                           Herzegovina
Ratko Magjarević   University of Zagreb, Croatia
Miroslav Končar   Oracle Healthcare Zagreb, Croatia
Almira Hadžović-Džuvo   University of Sarajevo, Bosnia and Herzegovina
Anne Humeau-Heurtier   University of Angers, France
Tamer Bego   University of Sarajevo, Bosnia and Herzegovina
Leandro Pecchia   University of Warwick, UK
Dušanka Bošković   University of Sarajevo, Bosnia and Herzegovina
Paulo Carvalho   University of Coimbra, Portugal
Jasmin Azemović   International Burch University, Bosnia and
                           Herzegovina

Contents

Posters (Short Papers)

Main Track (Full Papers)

Ecare@Home: A Distributed Research Environment on Semantic Interoperability

Amy Loutfi[1(✉)], Arne Jönsson[2], Lars Karlsson[1], Leili Lind[2], Maria Linden[3], Federico Pecora[1], and Thiemo Voigt[4]

[1] Örebro University, Örebro, Sweden
{amy.loutfi,lars.karlsson,federico.pecora}@oru.se
[2] SICS East, Linköping, Sweden
{arne.jonsson,leili.lind}@sics.se
[3] Mälardalen University, Västerås, Sweden
maria.linden@mdh.se
[4] SICS ICT, Stockholm, Sweden
thiemo.voigt@sics.se

Abstract. This paper presents the motivation and challenges to developing semantic interoperability for an internet of things network that is used in the context of home based care. The paper describes a research environment which examines these challenges and illustrates the motivation through a scenario whereby a network of devices in the home is used to provide high-level information about elderly patients by leveraging from techniques in context awareness, automated reasoning, and configuration planning.

Keywords: Semantic interoperability · Configuration planning · Health and care · Internet of Things

1 Introduction

A current vision in the area of ICT-supported independent living of the elderly involves populating the home with connected electronic devices ("things") such as sensors and actuators and linking them to the Internet. Creating such an Internet-of-Things infrastructure (IoT) is done with the ambition to provide automated information gathering and processing on top of which e-services can be built for the elderly residing in their homes [1]. Technically speaking IoT is mainly supported by continuous progress in wireless sensor/actuator networks software applications and by manufacturing low cost and energy efficient hardware for device communications. However, there is still the major the major challenge for expanding generic IoT technologies to efficient ICT-supported services for the elderly. Namely, services such as the personal health record (PHR) and other computerized "things" such as care and health related information resources, i.e., electronic health records (EHR), home-service (in Swedish: hemtjänst) documentation, end-user generated information, informal care-givers

© ICST Institute for Computer Sciences, Social Informatics and Telecommunications Engineering 2016
M.U. Ahmed et al. (Eds.): HealthyIoT 2016, LNICST 187, pp. 3–8, 2016.
DOI: 10.1007/978-3-319-51234-1_1

related information (e.g., information provided from family, neighbors, social networks etc.) must be integrated with the IoT infrastructure.

Ecare@home is a distributed research environment whose aim is to address the above vision by (1) performing research on selected fundamental issues in semantic interoperability with a particular focus on human-machine interoperability, that is to say how to enable users to query and control the IoT infrastructure on meaningful terms that are human interpretable and EHR/PHR compatible; and (2) testing the research results on a technical platform which is embedded in the Internet of Things and provides information with an unambiguous, shared meaning across IoT devices, elderly residents, relatives, health-and-care professionals and organizations and various personal information repositories and the various electronic health records associated with those.

This paper describes the main motivations and challenges which the research environment will address. It provides a brief overview of the various types of interoperability and then follows the main challenges that will be addressed within the scope of the research environment. A short scenario and illustrative scenario is outlined to conclude the paper.

2   The Dimensions of Interoperability

Generally speaking, interoperability is "the ability of two or more systems or components to exchange data and use information". Interoperability is a major concern of many organizations, including the European Commission which lists interoperability as a pillar in the Digital Agenda for Europe. This definition provides many challenges on how to (1) Get the data/information (2) Exchange data/information, and (3) Use the data/information in understanding it and being able to process it. There are different types of interoperability: technical, syntactical, semantic, and organizational. E-care@home focusses on semantic interoperability, still the planned research is expected to also impact the other types.

Semantic interoperability is seen as a key requirement for gaining the benefits of computerization of the health domain and much effort has been invested by both national programs and academia to understand and provide solutions for the problem of achieving semantic interoperability. Semantic interoperability is usually associated with the meaning of content, information or data, and concerns both the human and machine interpretation of content [3]. The focus here is on the semantic annotation of the data (for example, with domain knowledge) which can provide machine-interpretable descriptions on what the data represents, and meta-data such as where it originates from, how it can be related to its surroundings, what is providing it, and what are the quality, technical, and non-technical attributes. This semantic interpretation can be used for machine to machine communication (M2M). An example of M2M semantics-augmented communication would be a sensor measuring room temperature on demand of an end-user and, in relation to other information possibly available about the end-user, setting the temperature to an adequate level. Devices and sensors register through network gateway which writes their data into semantic database. Every time the sensor sends the temperature, the gateway writes it into the repository, and matches it with desired temperature inside the room where sensor is located. For example, the database could also keep information about the preferences of the user and contextual information needed to make room temperature decisions. However, another central aspect of semantic interoperability concerns the human interpretation of data and information provided by the IoT devices or by other humans respectively. Thus, interoperability on this level means that there is a common understanding between people and between people and devices of the meaning of the content being communicated. Regarding this type of interoperability E-care@home focuses on the contextualised semantic annotation of uncertain sensor/actuator data using symbolic reasoning methods. E-care@home also focuses on formal methods for modelling contextualised information from heterogeneous data sources so that a common understanding is achieved with the help of various mechanisms studied in the project, for instance ontology alignment. Ontologies not only provide some level of semantic expressiveness to the information they also allow the information exchange between applications and between different levels of abstraction.

The E-care@home research environment is needed to address an evitable and emerging challenge in sensor deployment in home and health environments. In short, this challenge entails adding value of raw sensor data by understanding the meaning of this data and involves collection, modelling, reasoning and distribution of context in relation to sensor data.

3   Semantic Modelling and Ontologies

Ontologies are tools for specifying the semantics of terminology systems in a well defined and unambiguous manner. Ontologies are used to improve communication either between humans or computers by specifying the semantics of the symbolic apparatus used in the communication process. The domain of application, here the health domain, is often significantly more complex than what practically usable ontologies might express. E.g. common health domain use cases require second-order reasoning which is not available in, e.g., any of the OWL profilesvii. Typically, use cases' requirements have to be balanced with computational effectiveness requirements and approximate solutions have to be developed and maintained. Thus, large-scale biomedical ontologies, such as SNOMED CT and NCI Thesaurus, are often using low-expressivity logics to allow to perform little reasoning, while smaller ontologies might allow higher expressivity. For enabling interoperability, all applications and users must share a common terminology. If an application uses a terminology different from another then a mapping between different ontologies must be made. A challenge is that in an care setting with an Iot infrastructure, the types of ontologies currently available are still disparate: on one hand, there is a growing establishment of ontologies for describing sensors and their observations such as the SSN; on the other hand, there are the ontologies in the health domain that capture relations between medical terms providing codes, terms, synonyms and definitions used in clinical documentation and reporting. Thus, there is a need to study these ontologies in a holistic context, e.g., a network of ontologies by reusing existing ones and alignments between those.

4   Context Reasoning in an Ecare@Home Setting

Ontologies and other semantic technologies can be key enabling technologies for sensor networks because they will improve semantic interoperability and integration, as well as facilitate reasoning and classification. Still, significant effort has yet to be placed on how to integrate the information in ontologies or other semantic models with formal reasoning methods specifically for improved sensor interpretation/annotation. Some work to this effect has been discussed in [Barghani et al.]. The domains considered so far deal with e.g. weather data where rule-based reasoning is relatively straight forward. Integrating proper reasoning techniques in more complex domains such as the one envisioned in Ecare@home is a more difficult problem. Sensors can only measure limited physical phenomenon and sensor data is inherently uncertain. Therefore, eventual reasoning methods must be also contending with the uncertain nature of the sensor data [2]. Context and patient profiling also plays a crucial role, and therefore the reasoner should make use of contextual information in a meaningful way. Finally, trust in the system is crucial for uptake, and enabling trust is often done via transparency, thus requiring explication and readability of the reasoner's output. Given these requirements, E-care@home will explore reasoning techniques e.g. answer set programming, for semantic-web data, focusing in particular on abductive reasoning methods that are non-monotonic in nature [4]. In part this has been examined in limited contexts of smart home networks, but including diverse semantic models as mentioned above is still a remaining challenge.

5   Semantic Interoperability for Service Discovery

Semantic interoperability not only enables a Machine-to-Human interaction but also enables a Human-to-Machine interaction, where in this case, human requests for services can transcend to machine readable code. High-level tasks requested by users such as "measure physical activity" should lead to a number of services being activated which also may relate to a number of devices which should provide the necessary data. In E-care@home we choose to see service composition as a configuration planning problem where configuration planning generates a functional configuration of a networked system consisting both of sensors and actuators distributed in the environment that solves a given task. In a functional configuration, sensory, computational and motoric functionalities belonging to the different devices are connected with communication channels. Another related and complementary area is web service composition. Web service composition, while not directly involving physical sensors and actuators, is concerned with ways of interconnecting selfcontained, self-describing, modular applications that can be published, located, and invoked across the web. A composite service is a set of services and the control and data flow among them. A number of approaches have been explored, from genetic algorithms, to neo-classical planning, and semantic information is often used for representing the domain. The challenge investigated in an E-care@home domain is to develop methods for service composition that not only fulfill hard constraints but also take into account preferences. Solving this challenge means that requests and queries can reconfigure device networks, thus adding robustness and reliability to obtaining information [6].

6   Testbeds and Scenario

An important objective of E-care@home is to evaluate the developed methods in real contexts. This includes a number of living lab environments but also as the environments progress we will include real test bed environments (e.g., IoT enhanced homes) where such test beds enable reliable data collection. For this objective to be met, synergies between existing projects and test beds will be made. Also, in order to properly verify results, test homes will be selected by first forming adequate use cases which outline the requirements for each test site and test persons involved in the evaluation. Figure 1 revisits the scenario outlined with respect to the above scientific objectives. In this Figure, a healthcare professional may want to query for specific information. This query probes one or several service(s) where the service requires that a particular configuration of devices in the home is active. If certain sensors were not activated (not shown in this example) they could be actuated by the configuration planner. Also the configuration planner takes into account preferences and not only hard constraints. To derive answers to queries or to infer information, the reasoning

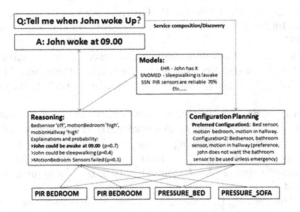

Fig. 1. An illustrative scenario which highlights the various challenges and motivations in achieving a semantic intereroperability between an IoT network and the various types of users in a home-based care setting.

module uses information both from the sensors (and eventual signal processing) as well from the models to contextualize the interpretation. Multiple explanations are generated and in particular, sensor uncertainties are factored into the final output. This example is illustrative but emphasizes an important aspect - that semantic AI techniques can be used to automate processes that configure, infer, and manage knowledge emerging from the sensor/actuator devices and, provide a meaningful output of the entire system.

7   Conclusion

This discussion paper presented a research environment Ecare@home whose objective is to rely on an IoT framework in order to gather information about inhabitants, abstract that information, and communicate it in a human consumable way to the various users of the system. Thus in E-care@home we aim to achieve something very different from the previous works in context-aware IoT and we aim to shift focus from network centric context awareness to data centric context awareness. The IoT notion is still very important as it is the setting for which the E-care@home domain exists. However, what is important in E-care@home is the data, observations and measurements and not the node that provides it. E-care@home embedded in an IoT will go beyond state of the art by bringing data-centric approach to IoT. Focus is put on interpretation of data, which is, translating sensor data to knowledge that is usable by people, organisations and applications. This involves abstraction whereby low-level data is converted to high-level knowledge and where prior knowledge and reasoning can interpret the data and infer beyond that which is physically measured.

References

1. Perera, C., Zaslavsky, A., Christen, P., Georgakopoulos, D.: Context aware computing for the Internet of Things: a survey. IEEE Commun. Surv. Tutorials J. **16**, 414–454 (2013)
2. Riboni, D., Bettini, C.: Context-aware activity recognition through a combination of ontological and statistical reasoning. In: Zhang, D., Portmann, M., Tan, A.-H., Indulska, J. (eds.) UIC 2009. LNCS, vol. 5585, pp. 39–53. Springer, Heidelberg (2009)
3. Kalra, D.: Barriers, approaches and research priorities for semantic interoperability in support of clinical care delivery. SemanticHEALTH deliverable 4.1
4. Alirezaie, M., Loutfi, A.: Reasoning for improved sensor data interpretation in a Smart Home. In: ARCOE-Logic 2014, International Workshop on Acquisition, Representation and Reasoning about Context with Logic, Linkoping, Sweden, 24–25 November 2014
5. Baldauf, M., Dustdar, S., Rosenberg, F.: A survey on context aware systems. Int. J. Ad Hoc Ubiquitous Comput. **2**(4), 263–277 (2007)
6. Silva-Lopez, L., Broxvall, M., Loutfi, A., Karlsson, L.: Towards conguration planning with partially ordered preferences: representation and results. KI-Künstliche Intelligenz **29**(2), 173–183 (2015)

Halmstad Intelligent Home - Capabilities and Opportunities

Jens Lundström[1,3]($\boxtimes$), Wagner O. De Morais[1,3], Maria Menezes[1],
Celeste Gabrielli[2], João Bentes[1], Anita Sant'Anna[1], Jonathan Synnott[2],
and Chris Nugent[1,2]

[1] Department of Intelligent Systems, Halmstad University,
Box 823, 301 18 Halmstad, Sweden
jens.lundstrom@hh.se
[2] School of Computing and Mathematics, University of Ulster, Jordanstown,
Shore Road, Newtownabbey, Co. Antrim BT37 0QB, UK
[3] HCH, Halmstad University, Box 823, 301 18 Halmstad, Sweden

Abstract. Research on intelligent environments, such as smart homes, concerns the mechanisms that intelligently orchestrate the pervasive technical infrastructure in the environment. However, significant challenges are to build, configure, use and maintain these systems. Providing personalized services while preserving the privacy of the occupants is also difficult. As an approach to facilitate research in this area, this paper presents the Halmstad Intelligent Home and a novel approach for multi-occupancy detection utilizing the presented environment. This paper also presents initial results and ongoing work.

Keywords: Intelligent environments · Multi-occupancy detection

1 Introduction

Over the past three decades, the concept of smart homes has emerged. Smart homes are residences equipped with technical solutions to enhance the resident's comfort, safety, security, entertainment and to increase energy-efficiency. Recently, smart homes are being constantly promoted to support effective and efficient healthcare of ageing and disabled individuals living alone. Smart homes employ artificial reasoning mechanisms that take into account the current and past states of the environment and its occupants to learn and anticipate needs. In general, smart homes are challenging to build, configure, use and maintain. Smart home systems often require complex algorithms, which in turn have parameters that need testing and tuning before further *out-of-lab* deployments. As a consequence, to deliver robust smart homes, one needs to investigate and experiment with a variety of hardware and software (e.g. system architectures, machine

This work was supported by the Knowledge Foundation of Sweden, Grant Number 2010/0271. Invest Northern Ireland partially supported this project under the Competence Centre Program Grant RD0513853 Connected Health Innovation Centre.

© ICST Institute for Computer Sciences, Social Informatics and Telecommunications Engineering 2016
M.U. Ahmed et al. (Eds.): HealthyIoT 2016, LNICST 187, pp. 9–15, 2016.
DOI: 10.1007/978-3-319-51234-1_2

learning methods, reasoning/decision schemes, strategies for interaction) components.

It is argued in this paper that these challenges can be holistically met by the use of the proposed Halmstad Intelligent Home (HINT). The current capabilities and future opportunities and research directions of HINT are described.

There are numerous examples of world-wide smart home implementations which focus on health-related services. The MavHome [2] showed successful prediction of user actions enabling the home to act as an intelligent agent. Another early, yet important example is The Aware Home [4] providing methods and tools for increased awareness of residents location, orientation and behaviours. However, few of the past smart homes extend the focus to go beyond specific algorithms as well as using more advanced sensors (e.g. physiological sensors such as EEG) and implementing services to respond to situations requiring attention. HINT provide the means to address these extensions.

Moreover, this paper presents how HINT is used for the development of robust and novel algorithms for the detection of several individuals in the home (i.e. multi-occupancy (M-O) detection). Robustness of M-O algorithms are important because for commercial smart homes to accurately adapt to residents activity patterns and privacy preferences it is critical to assure that only the patterns of a single person are being used.

2 The Halmstad Intelligent Home

At the Halmstad University campus, HINT is a fully functional one-bedroom apartment of 50 m^2 built to provide researchers, students and industrial partners with a technology-equipped realistic home environment. The layout of the apartment is illustrated in Fig. 1. HINT is expected to facilitate experiments and studies within the areas of intelligent environments, Ambient Assisted Living (AAL), and social robots. HINT is expected also to facilitate longitudinal studies by allowing subjects to stay in the apartment for extended periods of time.

2.1 Capabilities and Opportunities

Research at HINT focus on (1) the intelligent interconnection and collective behaviour of a diverse set of network-enabled technologies, and (2) the mechanisms that make the pervasive infrastructure of the smart environments behave intelligently.

HINT has been equipped with more than 60 sensors, including one "smart home in a box" kit [1], to detect the current state of the environment and its occupants. Magnetic switches detect the opening/closing of doors (label 1 in Fig. 1). Contact/touch sensors are positioned in the sofa and under the seat cushion to detect occupancy (label 2 in Fig. 1). Passive infrared (PIR) sensors are positioned to detect motion or occupancy in the different areas (label 3 in Fig. 1). Magnetic switches detect the opening/closing of cabinet's doors and

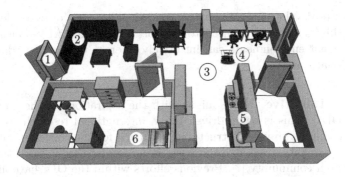

Fig. 1. The floor plan of HINT divided into multiple areas. Labels in the figure indicate capabilities.

drawers (label 5 in Fig. 1). Load-cells integrated into the bed frame measure weight and bed entrances and exits, and pressure sensitive sensors under the mattress detect vital signs (label 6 in Fig. 1). HINT has been built on top of a database-centric system architecture, meaning that the logic for the intelligent reactive and responsive behavior of the environment are implemented mostly within a database management system [3]. Following such an approach, HINT provides methods for: (1) physiological monitoring (e.g. vital signs) and safety monitoring and assistance (e.g. automatic lights), (2) functional monitoring (e.g. learning behaviour patterns and detecting deviating activities) [5], (3) emergency detection and response. To react and respond to events, HINT contains actuators. Motor actuators in the adjustable bed enable different bed positions to be selected (label 6 in Fig. 1). A vacuum cleaner-like robot (label 4 in Fig. 1) can navigate autonomously in the apartment and respond to detected anomalies, such as a fall.

Research at HINT is also focusing on technological solutions and seamless interfaces that are capable of recognizing and responding to the presence, health status and needs of residents in a unobtrusive and intuitive way. Although much progress has been made on developing wearable physiological sensors, and detecting and monitoring daily activities, research at HINT also aims to identify and respond to the resident's emotional state. Brain-Computer Interface (BCI) technologies are being currently investigated and will soon be integrated with existing capabilities of HINT to allow sensor fusion with existing sensors for an interpretation of emotional state. Furthermore, the resident's autonomy and participation in social life can be increased if the services are provided out of the home boundaries. Although some approaches have been proposed already [6], additional research is required to develop a middleware that supports self-adaptive systems, which can automatically discover and setup resources and facilitate continuous provisioning of services. Understanding an individual's emotional state is an important step in determining their needs. Consequently, one of the overarching goals of HINT is to develop and validate computational models of user affect using neurophysiological signals. At HINT we use BCI and Affective Computing technologies to develop and validate computational models of user affect. Subsequently, this model will be used to support accessible AAL applications in which intelligent environments can intuitively interact with users, adapting to their emotional state.

Open Data Initiative. HINT aligns with the aspirations of the Open Data Initiative (ODI). This is being driven by an international research consortium which is striving to provide a structured approach for the collection and annotation of high quality annotated data sets in an format that is easily accessible by the research community [7]. Previous efforts within the ODI have also been directed towards the generation of simulated datasets. There is, however, an opportunity to further progress the development of protocols for common data collection in addition to a suite of on-line tools for sharing and curating data, algorithms and results.

3   Showcase: Multi-occupancy Detection

To demonstrate the usefulness of HINT the development of an algorithm for M-O detection is described. M-O detection is referred to in this paper as the binary classification of the presence of more than one person in the home, at the same instance in time. The task of mapping sequences of events to the classification of the presence of one person or more is less studied than other tasks (e.g. *activity recognition*) and could be considered as challenging due to the following reasons: (A) Detection methods based solely on collected data may result in inaccuracies when residents perform previously unseen activities, not representative in training data. (B) Methods relying on training data where labels are collected from ground truth require tedious manual work to acquire. (C) The number of combinations of sensor events unfolds exponentially with the number of rooms, sensors, residents and potential activities. Therefore, to manually create programmatic rules is a difficult, time consuming and complex task which makes data-driven approaches favourable, however, challenging. Earlier approaches considered these challenges often by learning standard behaviour from the data. A common application concerns energy conservation in multi-resident buildings such as the work by Yang et al. [8]. Their approach targets occupancy modelling in an office environment where the problem is treated as a multi-class estimation where up to ten classes (meaning an environment occupied with nine individuals) were considered. The results illustrated that decision trees performed most accurately compared to alternative methods such as artificial neural networks. A significant difference between HINT and the environment used by Yang et al. is that a more rich sensor setup, e.g. sensors capturing $CO2$ and humidity was used by Yang et al. whereas in this study only PIR sensors, magnetic switches and pressure sensors were used. Such sensors can be considered to be more of standard sensor technology and often used in the context of capturing activities of daily lives.

Data: Events from participants occupying space, χ. Sequence of events, ψ, to predict as space occupancy. Sensor distances, J.

Result: Predictions of occupancy, ω.

1 $\alpha \leftarrow$ ExtractFeatures(χ);
2 $\beta \leftarrow$ CombineFeatures(α);
3 rf $\leftarrow$ TrainRandomForest($[\alpha,\ \beta]$, *labels*);
4 pred$_{RF}$, ambiguities $\leftarrow$ PredictMultOccByRF(rf, ExtractFeatures(ψ));
5 pred$_J$ $\leftarrow$ PredictMultOccByJ(J, ExtractTiming(ψ), thresh_probability);
6 **while** *next prediction and ambiguity is not empty* **do**
7 | **if** *J prediction is not M-O* **then**
8 | | **if** *ambiguity > thresh_ensemble_σ^2* **then**
9 | | | add (J) prediction to ω;
10 | | **else**
11 | | | add (RF) prediction to ω;
12 | | **end**
13 | **else**
14 | | add (J) prediction to ω;
15 | **end**
16 **end**

Algorithm 1. Algorithm for Multi-Occupancy Detection.

This paper describes, to the best of our knowledge a new approach to M-O detection using a combination of a classifier-based (Random Forest) and prior knowledge-based approach which eliminates the tedious data collection of M-O data (B) in addition to the need for creating manual rules (C). Training data for S-O observations (class one) is collected and combined in order to create the second class (M-O observations). To address the challenge with unseen patterns (A) the confidence of the classifier is weighted against the likelihood of sensor activations relative to their distance to each other, i.e. if the occurrence of two sensor events are *physically unlikely* then raise an M-O detection event.

3.1 Algorithm and Data Collection

The algorithm is designed to monitor when ambiguities are present in the data-driven methodology by following the variance of tree predictions in the forest (line 6 in Algorithm 1) and to adjust the system confidence in the data-driven model accordingly, i.e. less confidence in the data-driven model initiates a switch to the model based on prior knowledge (sensor distances, J). Features are represented as a simple count of events for each sensor triggered during a time window of 60 s as well as the last state of each sensor giving a total of 78 features per observation. The S-O dataset are combined (to create M-O dataset) by a summation of the count features as well as using the combined last state of two observations.

The data collection was performed by asking 10 participants to follow a protocol consisting of guidelines to eight activities: *go to bed, use bathroom, prepare breakfast, leave house, get cold drink, office work, get hot drink* and *prepare dinner*. The guidelines were written in a simplified form in order to provide participants with the freedom to perform an activity with a natural variation. All the participants were requested to sign an informed consent prior to the start of experiments. J, was compiled manually using measurements from a CAD-drawing of HINT and used with an assumed average in-door gait speed of $2\,m/s$ to compute the probability of two sensors events being likely to be triggered by a single person. The exponential cumulative distribution function was used to model this probability. The algorithm was tested by collecting data at HINT from additional two participants that performed various activities (both according to the protocol but also activities not found in the training data), in total 30 min was collected and contains both M-O and S-O observations.

3.2 Algorithm Results

A ROC curve created by varying the threshold for the tree prediction output variance (*thresh_ensembles_σ^2*) as well as varying the threshold for the probability of gait velocities (*thresh_probability*) can be seen in Fig. 2. A true positive (TP) is regarded as the correct classification of a M-O event. The combination of the data-driven and prior knowledge-driven approach shows the benefit of combining the two classifiers. Besides TP and FP rates the classifiers individually show accuracies of 82% (prior knowledge-based), 75% (Random Forest), and encouraging 96% using the proposed approach.

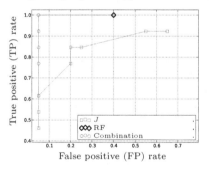

Fig. 2. ROC curve depicting TP/FP rates over the classifiers based on prior knowledge (squares), data (diamond) as well as the combination (circles).

4 Conclusions

This work presents capabilities and opportunities of the research environment HINT. One of the main goals of HINT is to facilitate algorithm development. The experience of the development of the proposed algorithm for M-O detection is that development time is significantly reduced when compared to designated tests in which environments have to be configured each time. Future work includes development of demonstrators able to showcase services (e.g. M-O detection) to a wider audience than researchers.

References

1. Cook, D.J., Crandall, A.S., Thomas, B.L., Krishnan, N.C.: CASAS: a smart home in a box. Computer **46**(7), 62–69 (2013)
2. Cook, D.J., Youngblood, G.M., Heierman III., E.O., Gopalratnam, K., Rao, S., Litvin, A., Khawaja, F.: MavHome: an agent-based smart home. In: PerCom, vol. 3, pp. 521–524 (2003)
3. de Morais, W.O., Lundström, J., Wickström, N.: Active in-database processing to support ambient assisted living systems. Sensors **14**(8), 14765–14785 (2014)
4. Kidd, C.D., et al.: The aware home: a living laboratory for ubiquitous computing research. In: Streitz, N.A., Siegel, J., Hartkopf, V., Konomi, S. (eds.) CoBuild 1999. LNCS, vol. 1670, pp. 191–198. Springer, Heidelberg (1999)
5. Lundström, J., Järpe, E., Verikas, A.: Detecting and exploring deviating behaviour of smart home residents. Expert Syst. Appl. **55**, 429–440 (2016)
6. Ma, S.P., Lee, W.T., Chen, P.C., Li, C.C.: Framework for enhancing mobile availability of RESTful services. Mobile Netw. Appl. **21**(2), 337–351 (2016)
7. Synnott, J., et al.: Environment simulation for the promotion of the open data initiative. In: 2016 IEEE International Conference on Smart Computing (SMART-COMP), pp. 1–6 (2016)
8. Yang, Z., Li, N., Becerik-Gerber, B., Orosz, M.: A systematic approach to occupancy modeling in ambient sensor-rich buildings. Simulation **90**(8), 960–977 (2014)

Healthcare Needs, Company Innovations, and Research - Enabling Solutions Within Embedded Sensor Systems for Health

Maria Lindén[✉], Therese Jagestig Bjurquist, and Mats Björkman

Embedded Sensor Systems for Health, Mälardalens Högskola,
Högskoleplan 1, 721 23 Västerås, Sweden
maria.linden@mdh.se

Abstract. This paper presents a research, innovation, and collaboration initiative at Mälardalen University in Sweden, within embedded sensor systems for health (ESS-H). ESS-H uses the needs of patients and caregivers as a starting point for identification of problems, and from this the development of new sensor systems to monitor elderly and/or multi-morbid people in their home is performed. The development of these systems is performed together with industry in order to enable innovations to reach the market in a near future. The initiative has during its first three years resulted in about 100 scientific publications. There are several research prototypes on their way to become commercial prototypes, and both the industry and healthcare are happy to continue the collaboration. The concept seems promising as a model to be used when aiming at developing new technologies for the healthcare sector.

Keywords: Embedded sensor systems for health · Health technology · Home monitoring

1 Introduction

The healthcare system in the western world is under change, challenged by demographic changes and people not only with one disease, but multi-morbid. The point-of-care is moving from hospitals to homes, a trend that is foreseen to increase in the future. This will empower the individual, in that he/she gets a larger influence over his/her health. Distributed health monitoring systems, comprising embedded sensor systems, will thus have a large potential market, nationally in Sweden as well as worldwide, and has the potential to be used both in the prevention of disease and in the monitoring and control of physiological states.

The costs and volumes of healthcare are increasing, mainly related to an aging population, and to the proliferation of multi-factorial diseases such as diabetes, stroke, chronic respiratory diseases, and heart disease. Intelligent and adaptive systems for the sensing and evaluation of health status for prevention, monitoring and rehabilitation are

---

Healthcare challenges addressed by researchers and industry in close collaboration.

© ICST Institute for Computer Sciences, Social Informatics and Telecommunications Engineering 2016
M.U. Ahmed et al. (Eds.): HealthyIoT 2016, LNICST 187, pp. 16–21, 2016.
DOI: 10.1007/978-3-319-51234-1_3

amongst the most important elements in resource-efficient and individualized health-care. Hence, the world market for products in the area of embedded sensor systems for health will grow tremendously in the decades to come.

The area of embedded sensor systems for health applications is rapidly developing, and there is a strong market pull for advanced intelligent sensor systems that strengthen or sustain the health of humans. Because of the rapid development and the market pull, research and product development is performed in parallel, and research results will be rapidly deployed in commercial products. The motivation from both a commercial and a scientific perspective is to be able to develop more capable and more dependable systems. From a commercial point of view, this means a competitive advantage. From a scientific point of view, this means contributing to an important area where the aims are to improve human health and minimize human suffering.

Embedded sensor systems for health is an important development and research area. The rapid development in physiological sensor and embedded systems technology gives possibilities for a broad deployment of sensor systems. This is an enabler for more intelligent and cognitive sensor systems; better informed systems as well as safer and more dependable systems, deployable in safety-critical applications (e.g. healthcare monitoring). To enable this, more efficient and predictable sensor nodes and communication techniques must be developed to match the development of the sensors themselves. This was one of the main challenges recognized by the EU ICT work program, FP7, and is also highlighted in Horizon 2020 [1]. For systems used in safety-critical applications, it is of uttermost importance that the behavior of the system and the dependability of the system can be tested and verified. Proper testing and verification of systems and system components will also enhance product quality and lower maintenance costs.

User friendliness, including intuitive use of the sensor systems, is essential in this application area, both with respect to safety and due to the fact that not all users (e.g. elderly and care staff) are familiar with this kind of technology. The involvement of users and focusing using their needs as a starting point in the development of new methods and systems is of large importance [2–8].

The aim of the present paper is to present a research, innovation, and collaboration initiative at Mälardalen University in Sweden, within embedded sensor systems for health (ESS-H). ESS-H uses the needs of the patients and caregivers as a starting-point for identification of problems, and from this, the development of new sensor systems to monitor elderly and/or multi-morbid people in their home is performed. The development of these systems is performed together with industry in order to enable innovations to reach the market in a near future.

2   Motivation

Changes in lifestyle, and increased expectations of a sustained high quality of life, also at higher ages, put new demands on our healthcare systems. To enable people to remain active, care providers need to provide wearable and distributed health monitoring systems, allowing people to continue their normal activities independent of location; at home, at work or in hospital. Monitoring of changes and trends in health status can facilitate early intervention and prevent severe conditions to develop. Hence, this can prevent suffering for patients and it also means large savings for society. Moving the point-of-care from hospitals to homes is a trend that will increase in the future. Distributed health monitoring systems will thus have a large potential market, nationally as well as worldwide.

Chronic diseases, such as heart diseases, stroke, cancer, chronic respiratory diseases and diabetes, were accounted for over 60% of all deaths in 2005 [9]. Further, 80% of premature heart disease, stroke and diabetes can be prevented with life-style changes [9]. The high prevalence of multi-morbidity makes the situation even more complicated, especially in older patients (a prevalence up to 98% has been observed) [10]. Monitoring health conditions related to multi-morbidity generates huge amounts of data, and methods to handle this information are called for. Further, a holistic approach must be considered. The situation is complex, since multiple diseases often interact with each other, and so can the medication. It is important to focus on the patient and to consider all diseases and interactions to give the best possible care for the patient.

Innovative development in medical technology and new medicines are predicted to have a large influence on future development of the health industry. It is predicted that 30% of the economical resources in the US will go to the health industry in the year 2050. Also the Swedish healthcare's share of the national budget, today 9% of the GNP, is predicted to increase due to an increasing demand on services that promote health-related quality of life [11].

The above needs and future market possibilities have drawn the attention of several of our industrial collaboration partners, as well as healthcare providers, e.g. Västmanland's county council and the municipality of Västerås. As a result of this, a cluster of health technology companies is identified.

3   Working Methods

The present research, innovation, and collaboration initiative within embedded sensor systems for health has several pillars that support the model. The collaboration with caregivers and presumptive end-users of the systems is crucial in order to identify the real needs. Research competence that can solve real problems and develop embedded sensor systems is just as important. Finally, the adoption of industrial partners in the project group is aimed at overcoming the common gap between research prototypes/solutions tested in project form and the final introduction into the market.

3.1   Identification of Needs and Challenges in Healthcare

Traditionally, development of new technology often has been technology driven, i.e. new technology has been introduced mostly because it is available. This is to a certain extend also true for the healthcare sector, and thus many systems have been introduced, which have not been based on actual request from the healthcare. Many of these technologies have anyhow meant a lot to healthcare, but still the spread might have been larger and even more successful if the starting point had been an actual need and request from the healthcare.

By including care staff, patients, relatives or workers, depending on the situations, throughout the whole development chain, the technology will be welcomed when ready to introduce in the care. Thus the researchers and also industrial partners need to collaborate closely with the healthcare by letting them take part in:

- the identification and formulation of the research problem
- finding possible solutions
- defining how the solution is working through test during the development and in its intended environment
- how the solution can be improved.

In the presented work, the healthcare staff has been involved during the continuous work. Further, the interest of new technology and solutions by the caregivers has facilitated the work. For example, in addition to our work, both the regional municipality Västerås stad and the county council Landstinget Västmanland have established their testbeds, inviting innovators and companies to meet their presumptive customers [12, 13].

The work has been performed by arranging focus groups, continuous discussions with presumptive users, and testing of prototypes together with the presumptive users.

3.2   Research Challenges

Dealing with human health and safety, it is extremely important that all parts of a sensor system for health fulfills both the aim for more capable systems as well as the aim for more dependable systems. Within ESS-H, research therefore is conducted with the aim of producing more capable systems, by advances in the core competence areas as will be explained below. The starting point is a real identified need from the caregivers, as explained above. Research is conducted with the aim to increase and verify dependability of new sensor systems.

ESS-H's core competence areas are:

- Biomedical Sensor Systems
- Biomedical Signal Processing
- Intelligent Decision Support
- Reliable Data communication.

Tasks that can be performed by an embedded sensor system for health includes acquisition of physiological parameters, different levels of signal processing of these parameters, data aggregation and data analysis, decision support, and feedback to both the patient an caregiver, adapted to the receiver.

Scientific challenges includes:

- Reliable acquisition of physiological data
- Personal biofeedback
- Reliable distribution of decision support
- Safe and secure communication (also considering personal integrity aspects).

3.3   Industrial Collaboration

Industrial partners have been included in the project as full members from the start of the initiative. Thus, they have been able to contribute to the solutions, and this also guarantees that the novel systems are possible to produce when they reach this phase. Some of the partner companies have also enrolled an employee as an industrial PhD student, which mean that this person actually can contribute to solve the research challenges together with the university staff. From the company perspective, this is a way to gain competence for their employees.

4   Result and Discussion

The interest from the healthcare sector to work together with the ESS-H researchers and industrial partners has been large. As starting point, identification of real problems that need to be addressed by the research team has been performed. When the research prototypes and industrial prototypes are developed (or before), there are two available testbeds which can identify further improvements of the systems from a user perspective This will hopefully also mean that the next step in the future, to introduce a system to the market, will be less cumbersome.

Bringing together academic and industrial researchers from several disciplines has shown to create a double cross-fertilization as a result of co-production. The cross-fertilization between academic and industrial researchers has been proven to increase the understanding of the problems at hand for all involved parties. Co-production will therefore lead to better results with better industrial value as well as higher academic importance. The cross-fertilization between disciplines is very important in systems-oriented research. Understanding of the whole system is important for obtaining the best solution for a particular subsystem. Without this system understanding, the risk of sub-optimization is apparent, if each discipline solves its sub-system problems without concerns about the overall system. Within the ESS-H projects, both types of cross-fertilization are present.

Presently, the initiative has been ongoing for three years, resulting in about 100 scientific publications. There are several research prototypes on their way to become commercial prototypes, and the industry is happy to continue and intensify the collaboration. Also the healthcare sector is happy to continue the collaboration in the present project and in new projects.

Acknowledgments. The present study was performed in the research profile ESS-H, financially supported by the Swedish Knowledge foundation.

References

1. Programme Horizon2020. https://ec.europa.eu/programmes/horizon2020/
2. De Rouck, S., Jacobs, A., Leys, M.: A methodology for shifting the focus of e-health support design onto user needs: a case in the homecare field. Int. J. Med. Inform. **77**(9), 589–601 (2008)

3. Clegg, C., Older Gray, M., Waterson, P.E.: The "charge of the byte brigade" and a socio-technical response. Int. J. Hum Comput Stud. 52(2), 235–251 (2000)
4. Holt, R., Makower, S., Jackson, A., Culmer, P., Levesley, M., Richardson, R.A.C., Mon Williams, M., Bhakta, B.: User involvement in developing rehabilitation robotic devices: an essential requirement. In: Proceedings of the 2007 IEEE 10th International Conference on Rehabilitation Robotics, 12-15 June, Noordwijk, The Netherlands (2007)
5. Kujala, S., Kauppine, M., Lehtola, L., Kojo, T.: The role of user involvement in requirements quality and project success. In: Proceedings of the 2005 13th IEEE International Conference on Requirements Engineering (RE 2005) (2005)
6. Hyysalo, S.: Predicting the use of a technology-driven invention. Eur. J. Soc. Sci. Res. 16(2), 117–137 (2003)
7. Kujala, S.: Early user involvement: a review of the benefits and challenges. Behav. Inf. Technol. 22(1), 1–16 (2003)
8. Sandberg, K., Jensen, L., Flø, R., Baldursdottir, R.K., Hurnasti, T.: Success stories of and barriers - user Involvement in development and evaluation of assistive technology. NUH Nordic Development Centre for Rehabilitation Technology (2001)
9. Preventing chronic diseases a vital investment, WHO GLOBAL REPORT. http://www.who.int/chp/chronic_disease_report/en/
10. Fortin, M., Bravo, G., Hudon, C., Vanasse, A., Lapointe, L.: Prevalence of multimorbidity among adults seen in family practice. Ann. Fam. Med. 3, 223–228 (2005). doi:10.1370/afm.272.59
11. Eliasson, G.: Svensk sjukvård som en framtida exportindustri? En industriekonomisk analys. Underlagsrapport nr 33 till Globaliseringsrådet. http://www.regeringen.se/sb/d/5146/a/124729
12. Västerås stad Mistel innovation. http://mistelinnovation.se/english/
13. Landstinget Västmaland Innovation. http://www.ltv.se/Forskningutbildning/Innovation/

A Case-Based Classification for Drivers' Alcohol Detection Using Physiological Signals

Hamidur Rahman[1(✉)], Shaibal Barua[1], Mobyen Uddin Ahmed[1],
Shahina Begum[1], and Bertil Hök[2]

[1] School of Innovation, Design and Engineering, Mälardalen University,
72123 Västerås, Sweden
hamidur.rahman@mdh.se
[2] Hök Instrument Ab, 72123 Västerås, Sweden

Abstract. This paper presents a case-based classification system for alcohol detection using physiological parameters. Here, four physiological parameters e.g. Heart Rate Variability (HRV), Respiration Rate (RR), Finger Temperature (FT), and Skin Conductance (SC) are used in a Case-based reasoning (CBR) system to detect alcoholic state. In this study, the participants are classified into two groups as *drunk* or *sober*. The experimental work shows that using the CBR classification approach the obtained accuracy for individual physiological parameters e.g., HRV is 85%, RR is 81%, FT is 95% and SC is 86%. On the other hand, the achieved accuracy is 88% while combining the four parameters i.e., HRV, RR, FT and SC using the CBR system. So, the evaluation illustrates that the CBR system based on physiological sensor signal can classify alcohol state accurately when a person is under influence of at least 0.2 g/l of alcohol.

Keywords: Physiological signals · Alcoholic detection · Case-based reasoning

1 Introduction

In the year 2012 in Sweden, 24% of car drivers were killed in crashes, under the influence of alcohol. Again 19% of road fatalities were due to intoxicated driver, rider, pedestrian, or cyclist. By the year 2020, Swedish government has a target that 99.9% of traffic should consist of drivers under the legal Blood Alcohol Content (BAC) limit of 0.2 g/l. [1]. Therefore, detection of alcoholic state of driver has been of great interest for car companies for many years.

A real time monitoring and detection of alcohol has been implemented using microwave sensor technology by Wendling et al. as described in [2]. Authors in [3] presented breathalyzer which is a device for estimating blood alcohol content (BAC) from breath sample. Also, Kiyomi et al. developed a new breath-suction type alcohol detector which does not require a long and hard blowing to the detector through a mouthpiece [4]. Another highly efficient system has been proposed with the aim at early detection and warning of dangerous vehicle maneuvers typically related to drunk driving [5]. Tunable Diode Laser Absorption Spectroscopy (TDLAS) based method for remote detection of alcohol concentration in vehicle has been suggested in [6].

© ICST Institute for Computer Sciences, Social Informatics and Telecommunications Engineering 2016
M.U. Ahmed et al. (Eds.): HealthyIoT 2016, LNICST 187, pp. 22–29, 2016.
DOI: 10.1007/978-3-319-51234-1_4

Kumar et al. proposed a real time non-intrusive drunk driver detection method using ECG sensors attaching under the driver seat [7]. A major limitation of the ECG sensor on the driver's seatback is very sensitive to impedance changes and disturbance resulted from environmentalnoise. K. Swathi et al. have compared and showed changes in the ECG features: heart rate, P wave, PR interval, QRS duration, QTC interval, ST segment, T wave, TP interval and frontal axis between non-alcoholics and alcoholics [8]. Kumar et al. have proposed a real time non-intrusive drunk driver detection method using ECG sensors attaching under the driver seat [9]. According to our knowledge, the research on drivers' alcoholic state classification based on physiological signals is very limited. However, future vehicles with embedded sensors in vehicles will get benefit from such systems.

In this paper, the proposed approach has considered 4 physiological parameters i.e., Heart Rate Variability (HRV), Respiration Rate (RR), Finger Temperature (FT), and Skin Conductance (SC). The Case-Based Reasoning (CBR) approach has been applied successfully in classification of physiological sensor signals [10–13].In addition, in some similar domains CBR has been achieved higher accuracy in classification compare to the other classification methods, such as Neural Network (NN) and Support Vector Machine (SVM) [14]. Here, the CBR approach is used as an artificial intelligence method to classify the alcoholic state of the driver. A number of features are extracted and selected to formulate a new query case, which is further entered into a case-library. The new case is matched with all previous cases and calculated a similarity value for each previous case. Based on the similarity value, most similar case together with its' class (i.e *drunk* or *sober*) is used for the final classification. An experiment work has been conducted, where the classification accuracy is observed considering both each individual parameters and as well as combination of them.

The rest of the paper is organized as follows: Sect. 2 describes materials and methods, and Sect. 3 presents results and evaluation. Finally, Sect. 4 summarizes the work.

2 Materials and Methods

2.1 Data Collection

The data have been collected from 12healthyparticipants (10 male, 12 female), age between 22 and 32 years. A total of five different sessions consisting 12 experiments were conducted where 3 sessions (6 tests) were taken place in normal lab environment in sitting position, one session (3 tests) was carried out using driving simulator, Häslö, Västerås[1] and another session (3 tests) was conducted in Mälardalen University robotics lab using Volvo construction equipment simulator called Volvo articulated hauler machine. Each participant has signed a letter of consent in order to participate in the study. The participants were informed about the study and the data acquisition sessions. In each session, two measurements were taken, without drinking alcohol i.e. the person is sober and when the test person is intoxicated with 37.5% of alcohol i.e.

---

[1] http://www.htop.se/start.asp?lang=1.

drunk. Each test subject was in a seated position and the physiological sensors data were collected with cStress[2] system attached to the subject's body. In order to detect how physiological parameters changes with blood alcohol concentration the alcohol level is acquired in every two minutes using Sesame alcohol measurement device[3] when the person has been intoxicated. Here, using the cStress system, in each session, five physiological parameters i.e., RR, IBI, FT, and SC were collected for each test person.

2.2   Approach

The overview of the proposed classification system is presented as a step diagram in Fig. 1. The 4 physiological signals that are obtained from each participant during data collection phase are inputted into the CBR system. Duration of recording for each participant is around 10 min. In order to get a homogeneous dataset, during the pre-processing step, the first and last one minute recording from each data set have been discarded, then 8 min recording have been considered for further processing. These 8 min signals are then segmented into 2 min data for the feature extraction. Before feature extraction from these segmented signals, noise and artifacts are handled for each individual signal. A k-nearest neighbor (K-NN) based interpolation algorithm has been applied to handle artifacts in IBI signals [15]; and Infinite impulse response (IIR) filter and smoothing running average method available in cStress system have been used to handle artifacts in FT, SC and RR signals. Thereafter, features are extracted from the segmented signals for all input signals. Then, using the extracted features, case formulation is performed and a case library is built for the CBR classification.

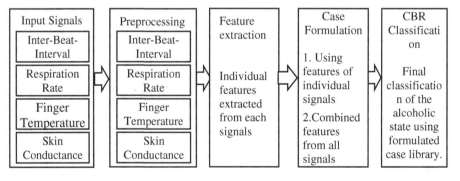

Fig. 1. Step diagram of the proposed CBR classification scheme.

2.2.1   Feature Extraction

Feature extraction is one of the important tasks to solve any classification problem using a classifier. A number of features for each parameter have been extracted. Here, both the time domain and frequency domain features of HRV have been extracted from the IBI signals. In time domain, statistical methods are applied on the Inter-beat-interval (IBI) signals to extract standard deviation of RR intervals (SDNN), root mean square of the all successive RR interval difference (RMSSD), number of pairs of adjacent NN intervals differing by more than 50 ms (NN50) features, percentage of NN50 count (pNN50), and standard deviation of differences between adjacent NN intervals (SDSD). To extract frequency domain features of HRV, power spectral density (PSD) has been estimated from the IBI Signal. Low frequency power (LF) (0.04–0.15 Hz), high frequency power (HF) (0.15–0.4 Hz), total power, LF peak (0.04–0.15 Hz), HF peak (0.15–0.4 Hz), and total peak are extracted from the PSD of IBI signal. Moreover, power at ultra-low frequency range (ULF) (≤ 0.003 Hz) power, very low frequency range (VLF) (0.003–0.04 Hz), normalized LF power (LF/(Total power − VLF)*100), and normalized HF power (HF/(Total power − VLF)*100) are estimated from the PSD. From the RR signal, arithmetic mean and standard deviation are calculated as features in time domain. Another feature called dominant respiration frequency (DRF) is estimated from the PSD of RR signal. DRF is the maximum energy frequency which lies between the frequency range 0.1 Hz and 1.5 Hz [16]. From FT and SC signals a derivative of slope is used to extract the important features [17]. In addition, mean, standard deviation, max, and temperatures are calculated from FT and SC as features. Different weight values in the range between 1 and 10 have been used to achieve optimal accuracy. The extracted and selected features from the 4 physiological signals and their optimal weight values for the CBR classification are presented in Table 2.

2.2.2   Case Formulation

In developing a CBR system, the first task is the case formulation, which represents the instance of things or a part of a situation that is experienced. A case library or case base has been constructed from the formulated cases where each case comprises unique features extracted from the 4 physiological sensor signals to describe a problem. In this study, here, each case is labeled as '*Sober*' or '*Drunk*' based on the recording events. Hence, CBR classification classifies each subjects as *Sober* or *Drunk* state. Moreover, during the case formulation two approaches were taken into consideration; 1st create a case base using the features extracted from each individual physiological parameters only i.e., HRV, RR, SC and FT only; 2nd, a case is formulated based on combination of features extracted from the individual physiological parameters.

2.2.3   CBR Classification

In CBR, the term 'case' represents an experience that is achieved from a previously solved problem; the term 'based' means in CBR cases are the source for reasoning; and the term 'reasoning' means the approach of problem solving i.e., the intension of CBR is to solve a problem by drawing conclusion using previously solved cases [18]. Aamodt and Plaza [19] have described the CBR cycle, which contains four steps that are *Retrieve, Reuse, Revise and Retain*. Here, in the proposed CBR classification system the first 3 phases are implemented.

In this study, previous solved cases are retrieved for a current query case using the similarity function presented in Eq. 1.

$$Similarity(T, S) = \sum_{i=1}^{n} W_i \times f(T_i, S_i) \tag{1}$$

Where T is the target or new case, S is retrieved cases stored in the case library, and f is the similarity function, and $W_i = \frac{lw}{\sum_{i=0}^{n} lw_i}$ and lw_i is a local weight for each feature. The weight for each features are gathered by the help of expert of the domain and presented in Table 1 (see Sect. 2.2.1 (Feature Extraction)). Euclidean distance function is used to calculate the similarity f of each feature by normalizing the absolute difference between two features for the current and retrieved cases and dividing that by the difference of the maximum and minimum distance. The similarity then gets by subtracts the result from 1, represented in Eq. 2. The similarity value '1' means 100% similar between two cases and the value '0' means dissimilar between the cases.

$$(T_i, S_i) = 1 - \frac{abs(T_i, S_i)}{max(T_i, S_i) - \min(T_i, S_i)} \tag{2}$$

For the classification of combined features, additional weights are considered for each type of signals based on the classification accuracy of each signals. Hence, Eq. 1 is updated by multiplying the weights value for each signal, which is shown in Eq. 3.

$$Similarity(T, S) = \sum_{i=1}^{n} W_i \times f(T_i, S_i) \times S_w \tag{3}$$

Here, S_w is the weight value for each signal based on their individual classification.

3   Results and Evaluation

The proposed approach is evaluated in two fold. First, an evaluation is performed for the cases considering features obtained from individual signals. Secondly, building cases by combining features from all four signals. In the combined approach, additional weight values are multiplied with the similarity function. The weight values are considered based on the evaluation result obtained in the first phase i.e., considering individual signals. For CBR classification, a number of different weight values ranges from 0 to 10 have been assigned to achieve maximum accuracy for each parameter and also for combined features.

Table 1 shows the accuracy for K1 considering the top most similar retrieved case; and for K2 considering the top 2 most similar cases are retrieved, where one of them matches with the target case. It can be seen form Table 1 that the highest accuracy considering K1 for HRV, FT, SC and RR is 67%, 89%, 67% and 59% and considering

K2 is 85%, 95%, 86% and 81% respectively. However, the accuracy for combination of all four features for K1 and K2 are 83% and 88% respectively.

Table 2 shows the summary of the evaluation. In total, 103 are cases labeled with either *Sober* or *Drunk* in combined. However, for individual HRV has 148, RR has 164, FT and SC have 119 cases for consideration. It can be seen from Table 3 that the sensitivity of the system is 81% for HRV, 78% for RR, 97% for FT, and 89% for SC. The specificity is 80% for HRV, 76% for RR, 82% for FT, and 81% for SC. Thus, the overall accuracy for HRV is 85%, RR is 81%, FT is 95% and SC is 86% respectively. Furthermore, for the cases while combining all the four parameters the obtained sensitivity is 83%, specificity is 92% and accuracy is 88%.

Table 1. A list of accuracy for individual and combined feature based classification for K1 and K2

	HRV		FT		SC		RR		Combination (HRV+FT+SC+RR)	
	K1	K2	K1	K2	K1	K2	0.56	0.81	K1	K2
Accuracy1	0.62	0.85	0.88	0.93	0.63	0.83	0.57	0.79	0.74	0.85
Accuracy2	0.60	0.84	0.89	0.94	0.67	0.86	0.57	0.79	0.74	0.84
Accuracy3	0.63	0.79	0.88	0.95	0.65	0.86	0.58	0.8	0.73	0.84
Accuracy4	0.59	0.79	0.88	0.95	0.63	0.86	0.58	0.81	0.74	0.83
Accuracy5	0.66	0.84	0.89	0.95	0.65	0.86	0.59	0.81	0.67	0.83
Accuracy6	0.65	0.84	0.88	0.94	0.67	0.85	0.58	0.81	0.65	0.83
Accuracy7	0.67	0.85			0.65	0.86	0.57	0.8	0.73	0.84
Accuracy8	0.63	0.85			0.65	0.87	0.55	0.74	0.75	0.85
Accuracy9	0.63	0.85			0.65	0.86	0.57	0.71	0.77	0.86
Accuracy10	0.63	0.82			0.64	0.83			0.80	0.85
Accuracy11									0.80	0.88
Accuracy12									0.80	0.87
Accuracy13									0.72	0.85
Accuracy14									0.79	0.87
Accuracy15									0.82	0.87
Accuracy16									0.83	0.88
Accuracy17									0.81	0.87
Accuracy18									0.83	0.87

Table 2. Classification of individual and combined features for K2

Feature	HRV	RR	FT	SC	Combined
Total case	148	164	119	119	103
P (Drunk Cases)	74	82	62	62	54
N (Sober Cases)	74	82	57	57	49
TP	60	64	60	55	45
FP	15	20	10	11	4
TN	59	62	47	46	45
FN	14	18	2	7	9
Sensitivity TP/(TP + FN)	0.81	0.78	0.97	0.89	0.83
Specificity TN/(FP + TN)	0.80	0.76	0.82	0.81	0.92
Accuracy (TP + TN)/(P + N)	0.85	0.81	0.95	0.86	0.88

4 Discussion and Summary

In this paper, a CBR classification system for driver's alcoholic state detection based on multiple physiological parameters (HRV, RR, FT and SC) and CBR has been proposed. Both the individual and combined signals have been classified using the CBR system and presented in Table 1. Here, FT has the highest sensitivity, Specificity and overall accuracy while RR has the lowest accuracy. Though FT has highest accuracy for individual signal classification but it could be biased by external factors. Therefore, combined classification has been conducted to achieve a more reliable result. It has been observed while combining the 4 physiological parameters, an acceptable accuracy has been achieved considering the sensitivity, Specificity and overall accuracy. Thus, the proposed approach for driver's alcoholic state classification shows one of the alternative of the Breathalyzer and it has significant potential for advancing many real time applications such as driver monitoring.

Acknowledgement. The authors would like to acknowledge the Swedish Knowledge Foundation (KKS), Hök instrument AB, Volvo Car Corporation (VCC), The Swedish National Road and Transport Research Institute (VTI), Autoliv AB, Prevas AB Sweden, Hässlögymnasiets, Västerås and all the test subjects for their support of the research projects in this area.

References

1. Road Safety Annual Report 2015. OECD Publishing, Paris, OECD/ITF (2015)
2. Wendling, L., Cullen, J.D., Al-Shamma'a, A., Shaw, A.: Real time monitoring and detection of alcohol using microwave sensor technology. In: 2009 Second International Conference on Developments in eSystems Engineering (DESE), pp. 113–116 (2009)
3. Rahim, H.A., Hassan, S.D.S.: Breathalyzer enabled ignition switch system. In: 2010 6th International Colloquium on Signal Processing and Its Applications (CSPA), pp. 1–4 (2010)
4. Sakakibara, K., Taguchi, T., Nakashima, A., Wakita, T., Yabu, S., Atsumi, B.: Development of a new breath alcohol detector without mouthpiece to prevent alcohol-impaired driving. In: IEEE International Conference on Vehicular Electronics and Safety (ICVES 2008), pp. 299–302 (2008)
5. Jiangpeng, D., Jin, T., Xiaole, B., Zhaohui, S., Dong, X.: Mobile phone based drunk driving detection. In: 2010 4th International Conference on-NO PERMISSIONS Pervasive Computing Technologies for Healthcare (PervasiveHealth), pp. 1–8 (2010)
6. Shao, J., Tang, Q.-J., Cheng, C., Li, Z.-Y., Wu, Y.-X.: Remote detection of alcohol concentration in vehicle based on TDLAS. In: 2010 Symposium on Photonics and Optoelectronic (SOPO), pp. 1–3 (2010)
7. Murata, K., Fujita, E., Kojima, S., Maeda, S., Ogura, Y., Kamei, T., et al.: Noninvasive biological sensor system for detection of drunk driving. IEEE Trans. Inf. Technol. Biomed. **15**, 19–25 (2011)
8. Swathi, K., Ahamed, N.: Study ECG effects in alcoholic and normals. J. Pharmaceutical Sci. Res. **6**, 263–265 (2014)
9. Kumar, V.V.: The Method for non-aggression biological signal sensing system of drinking detection. Int. J. Res. Sci. Eng. **1**, 60–61 (2008)

10. Ahmed, M.U., Begum, S., Funk, P., Xiong, N., Schéele, B.V.: A multi-module case based biofeedback system for stress treatment. Artif. Intell. Med. **51**(2), 107–115 (2011)
11. Begum, S., Ahmed, M.U., Funk, P., Xiong, N., Folke, M.: Case-based reasoning systems in the health sciences: a survey of recent trends and developments. IEEE Trans. Syst. Man Cybern. Part C Appl. Rev. **41**(4), 421–434 (2011)
12. Begum, S., Barua, S., Filla, R., Ahmed, M.U.: Classification of physiological signals for wheel loader operators using multi-scale entropy analysis and case-based reasoning. Expert Syst. Appl. **41**(2), 295–305 (2013)
13. Begum, S., Barua, S., Ahmed, M.U.: Physiological sensor signals classification for healthcare using sensor data fusion and case-based reasoning. Sensors **14**(7), 11770–11785 (2014). (Special Issue on Sensors Data Fusion for Healthcare)
14. Barua, S., Begum, S., Ahmed, M.U.: Supervised machine learning algorithms to diagnose stress for vehicle drivers based on physiological sensor signals. In: 12th International Conference on Wearable Micro and Nano Technologies for Personalized Health (2015)
15. Begum, S., Islam, M.S., Ahmed, M.U., Funk, P.: K-NN based interpolation to handle artifacts for heart rate variability analysis. In: 2011 IEEE International Symposium on Presented at the Signal Processing and Information Technology (ISSPIT) (2011)
16. Rigas, G., Goletsis, Y., Bougia, P.: Towards river's state recognition on real driving conditions. Int. J. Veh. Technol. (2011)
17. Begum, S., Ahmed, M.U., Funk, P., Xiong, N., Schéele, B.V.: A case-based decision support system for individual stress diagnosis using fuzzy similarity matching. Comput. Intell. **25**, 180–195 (2009)
18. Michael, M.R., Rosina, O.W.: Case-Based Reasoning: A Textbook, 1st edn. Springer, Heidelberg (2013)
19. Aamodt, A., Plaza, E.: Case-based reasoning: foundational issues, methodological variations, and system approaches. AI Commun. **7**, 39–59 (1994)

Towards a Probabilistic Method for Longitudinal Monitoring in Health Care

Ning Xiong$^{(\boxtimes)}$ and Peter Funk

School of Innovation, Design and Engineering,
Mälardalen University, 72123 Västerås, Sweden
{ning.xiong,peter.funk}@mdh.se

Abstract. The advances in IoT and wearable sensors enable long term monitoring, which promotes earlier and more reliable diagnosis in health care. This
position paper proposes a probabilistic method to address the challenges in
handling longitudinal sensor signals that are subject to stochastic uncertainty in
health monitoring. We first explain how a longitudinal signal can be transformed
into a Markov model represented as a matrix of conditional probabilities. Further, discussions are made on how the derived models of signals can be utilized
for anomaly detection and classification for medical diagnosis.

Keywords: Health monitoring · Longitudinal signal · Symbolic time series ·
Markov model · Case-based reasoning

1 Introduction

In recent years there has been rising interest in wearable sensors for personal health
care [1]. Integrating these devices with wireless communication provided by IoT [2] is
hopeful to create new technology that would have significant impact on the way
clinical monitoring is performed nowadays. Particularly IoT provides a convenient
means of transmitting and recording long term biological signals, which convey much
richer information than conventional lab-test based static measurements. Utilizing
dynamic longitudinal data is beneficial to promote earlier and more accurate diagnosis
results for future health monitoring systems.

However, longitudinal monitoring in health care faces two major challenges. The
first lies in the big data volume that is collected continuously. There is a gap between
the rate at which data become available and our ability to interpret and handle them. It
is crucial to develop novel data analysis and mining tools to extract concise information
and identify abnormality in real-time during the monitoring of the subject.

The second challenge arises from the inherently stochastic nature of data evolution
in health monitoring. It is important to characterize the truly dynamic property of
temporal patterns while ignoring random triviality in data analysis. How to represent
uncertain characteristics residing in data and how to utilize such uncertain information
in reasoning/learning is a key issue for reliable (anomaly) detection and diagnosis.

This position paper aims to suggests a probabilistic method to address the above
two challenges. The proposed roadmap consists of three consecutive stages. The first is
to convert original, real-valued signals into shorter symbolic time series. In the second

© ICST Institute for Computer Sciences, Social Informatics and Telecommunications Engineering 2016
M.U. Ahmed et al. (Eds.): HealthyIoT 2016, LNICST 187, pp. 30–35, 2016.
DOI: 10.1007/978-3-319-51234-1_5

stage, the converted time series data are further transformed into a concise matrix to capture the stochastic and dynamic property of the underlying process. Finally, in the third stage, different matrices (derived from original sensor signals) are compared with each other in order to detect significant change of data transition patterns as well as to identify possible health problems. We hope that the presented work would offer an initial step towards the development of a useful framework to tackle uncertain and longitudinal data profiles in health monitoring.

The remainder of the paper is as follows. Section 2 presents the ways in which a longitudinal signal can be modeled into a concise matrix. Section 3 discusses how such matrices can be utilized for anomaly detection and diagnosis in health monitoring. Finally, the paper is concluded in Sect. 4.

2 Concise Modeling of Longitudinal Signals

This section explains how a longitudinal signal can be compressed by a concise model. It is accomplished by the following two steps: (1) converting the original signal into a symbolic series; (2) modeling the symbolic series with a matrix of pattern transition probabilities.

2.1 Converting Signal into Symbolic Time Series

The first step in our solution is to convert the sampling-point based representation of the signal into an interval-based representation. An interval consists of a set of consecutive sampling points and thus it encompasses multiple sampling periods in the time dimension. Subsequently, data within an identical interval have to be generalized into one symbolic value; the symbolization is conducted via discretization of the range of possible values of the signal. Next we shall outline three approaches that can be used in practice to convert a primary numerical signal into a shorter time series profile.

Symbolic Approximation was proposed in [3], in which the whole duration of the signal is divided into equally sized intervals, i.e., each interval encompasses the same amount of sampling periods. The data in each interval is averaged into a mean value, thereby creating an intermediate sequence of real numbers summarizing signal behaviors in the consecutive time intervals. This sequence is termed as PAA (Piecewise Aggregate Approximation) of the original signal. Then the PAA sequence is further transformed into a symbolic form by mapping the real numbers in it into corresponding symbols.

Temporal Abstraction [4, 5] was proposed to derive high level generalization of data from time-stamped representations towards interval-based interpretations. Basically this is achieved by aggregating adjacent entities falling in the same region into a cluster and summarizing behaviors in this cluster with a concept (symbol) corresponding to the region. Thereafter, arranging concepts of clusters according to the order of their appearances produces a required symbolic time series.

More specifically, the tasks of temporal abstraction can be performed on state abstraction or trend abstraction. The former focuses on the measured values themselves to extract intervals associated with qualitative concepts such as low, normal, and high, while the latter focuses differences between two neighboring records to discover patterns of changes such as increase, decrease, and stationarity in the series. Obviously trend abstraction is equivalent to applying state abstraction to the secondary series of differences derived from the primary signal of measurements.

Alternatively, symbolic time series can also be obtained via **Phase-Based Pattern Identification**, as suggested in [6]. It is motivated by the fact that sometimes a lengthy sensor signal from health monitoring may comprise a series of phases and every phase has its importance to identify its property (pattern) alone. In such cases, we need to separate the profile of the signal into a set of sub-signals with each of which corresponding to a phase inside the whole duration. As sub-signals are shorter and simpler, it would be relatively easy to classify their patterns using traditional signal processing and machine learning approaches. The final symbolic series is constructed by combining the patterns of sub-signals in terms of the order of appearance, which provides a compact and abstract representation of the evolution of data in the whole signal profile.

2.2   Characterization as Markov Model

After conversion of the primary signal as stated in Subsect. 2.1, we acquire a symbolic time series $x(1)$, $x(2)$, ..., $x(t)$, ..., $x(n)$, in which an element $x(t) = S_i$ reflects the fact that the process under monitoring is in state (symbol) S_i at time step t. We have to focus on transitions of states between adjacent time steps rather than single symbolic values for characterizing the evolution of data in the time series.

Since this time series originates from a stochastic process in health monitoring, we suggest using the Markov model to depict the uncertain transitions in it. According to the Markov property, the probability for the state at time step $t + 1$ is only dependent on the state at time step t, regardless of the states in the previous time steps, i.e.,

$$P\{x(t+1) = S_j | x(t) = S_i, x(t-1) = S_k, \cdots\} = P\{x(t+1) = S_j | x(t) = S_i\} \quad (1)$$

Equation (1) implies that only transitions between two successive time steps are required in the model of the symbolic time series.

Let $\{S_1, S_2, ..., S_M\}$ be the set of possible states (symbols) of the process monitored for health care. We use a_{ij} $(i, j = 1, 2, ..., M)$ to denote the probability for the process to move from state S_i to state S_j in two consecutive time steps. Hence a_{ij} is defined as a conditional probability:

$$a_{ij} \equiv P\{x(t+1) = S_j | x(t) = S_i\} \quad \forall t \quad (2)$$

This conditional probability in Eq. (2) can simply be calculated as the ratio of the number of transitions from state S_i to S_j to the number of transitions starting from S_i in the series.

Finally, the stochastic Markov model of the symbolic time series can be formulated as a concise matrix as follows:

$$G = \begin{pmatrix} a_{11} & a_{12} & \cdots & a_{1M} \\ a_{21} & a_{22} & \cdots & a_{2M} \\ \cdots & \cdots & \cdots & \cdots \\ a_{M1} & a_{M2} & \cdots & a_{MM} \end{pmatrix} \tag{3}$$

with $a_{ij} \geq 0$ and $\sum_{j=1}^{M} a_{ij} = 1 \quad \forall i$

where the elements in row i reveal the probability distribution for the next state after state S_i. Note that the size of the matrix is merely determined by the number of states (or symbols), which is independent of the length of the time series. This offers an attractive opportunity of strong data reduction to benefit data storage and handling in the health monitoring system.

3 Anomaly Detection and Diagnosis

This section addresses how the model of the symbolic time series can be utilized for anomaly detection and diagnosis in health monitoring. First we shall explain the the ways of calculating the distance between matrices of time series in Subsect. 3.1. Then, in Subsect. 3.2, we discuss how the developed distance metric can be employed to support detection and classification of abnormal situations.

3.1 Measuring the Distance Between Two Models

Our goal is to evaluate the distance between two symbolic time series cases that are represented by matrices G and G' respectively. As each row in these matrices represents a distribution of probabilities of state transition, we first calculate the distances for pairs of probability distributions from the two matrices. Then the distances between probability distributions for various starting states are aggregated to achieve an overall dissimilarity between the two models of time series.

The matching of two probability distributions can be performed in terms of relative entropy or information gain. Hence we apply Jeffreys divergence (J-divergence) [7] to quantitatively distinguish two probability distributions in comparison. Suppose that $TB(i) = [a_{i1}, a_{i2}, \cdots, a_{iM}]$ and $TB'(i) = [a'_{i1}, a'_{i2}, \cdots, a'_{iM}]$ are two probability distributions described in the ith rows of G and G' respectively, the J-divergence between $TB(i)$ and $TB'(i)$ is formulated as follows:

$$\begin{aligned} J(TB(i), TB'(i)) &= \sum_{j=1}^{M} a_{ij} \cdot log\left(\frac{a_{ij}}{a'_{ij}}\right) + \sum_{j=1}^{M} a'_{ij} \cdot log\left(\frac{a'_{ij}}{a_{ij}}\right) \\ &= \sum_{j=1}^{M} \left(a_{ij} - a'_{ij}\right) \cdot log\left(\frac{a_{ij}}{a'_{ij}}\right) \end{aligned} \tag{4}$$

For acquiring the overall distance between matrices (representing the time series), the values of J-divergence on different probability distributions have to be combined.

If we deem probability distributions for various starting states are equally important, we can simply average the J-divergence values derived from every pair of probability distribution in G and its counterpart in G'. Otherwise, we can define the weighted average of the J-divergence values as the final distance metric, where the weights reflect the importance of different probability distributions.

Further, the weights for the probability distributions can be determined automatically from a set of time series models (matrices) with known classes. Our idea, inspired from the work in [8], is that we retrieve the nearest models using a single J-divergence index and then we base the quality of retrieved models to assess the importance of the probability distribution, on which the J-divergence value is derived. More concretely, for every model in the collection, a set of nearest models are retrieved in terms of the J-divergence to yield a local alignment degree for that model. Secondly, the global alignment degree is calculated as the mean of the local alignment degrees for all models in the collection. Finally, the global alignment degree is assigned as the weight to the probability distribution in inspection.

3.2   Distance-Based Decisions

The distance metric developed for time series models can be used for two purposes. The first is to detect significant deviation of data evolution during the monitoring process (anomaly detection). The second is to further identify the class of the abnormal situation (if anomaly is detected) for medical diagnosis.

The anomaly detection can be made by comparing the model of time series in the latest time window with that of the preceding window. If the distance between them is sufficiently large, it indicates a potential abnormality since the probabilities of sate transitions have changed significantly in the new time window. Of course, the size of the window is an important parameter that affects the results of monitoring. One heuristic to find a proper value for that parameter would be gradually increasing the window size until the matrix of the time series becomes stable. Discovering optimal window sizes for different phases of the signal may improve anomaly detection.

For identification of the class of an abnormal situation, we advocate the application of case-based reasoning (CBR) which has been proved as a powerful methodology to solve new problems by learning from previous experiences [9]. CBR is based on the principle that similar problems have similar solutions. Therefore, given an abnormal time series in the latest window, we measure the distances of its matrix and the classified models (of time series) in the case library. The nearest models are thereby retrieved, and we resort to the classes of the retrieved models as the foundation to predict the class of the new abnormal situation. Feature selection [10] is sometimes needed here to identify the most important elements of the models for comparison, and fuzzy rule-based matching [11] can support more flexible criteria for assessment of the discrepancy between two time series models.

4 Conclusion

This paper puts forward a probabilistic method to deal with large data volumes in long term monitoring in health care. The key in our work lies in the conversion of longitudinal signals into shorter symbolic time series as well as depicting the stochastic property of the symbolic series with a Markov model. As the size of the Markov model only is related to the number of patterns rather than the length of the signal, it contributes with a big reduction of the data that needs to be stored and processed. We also illustrate that the Markov models derived from primary signals can be conveniently utilized to detect and classify abnormality in signals during the monitoring process.

However, it should be admitted that Markov models only consider the current state information. In the future work we are going to extend the current model to accommodate historical and contextual information to enable diagnosis and reasoning of higher accuracy.

Acknowledgement. This research is carried out within the research profile "Embedded Sensor Systems for Health", funded by the Knowledge Foundation of Sweden.

References

1. Pantelopoulos, A., Bourbakis, N.: A survey on wearable sensor-based systems for health monitoring and prognosis. IEEE Trans. Sys. Man Cybern. Part C Appl. Rev. **40**, 1–12 (2010)
2. Milenkovi, A., Otto, C., Jovanov, E.: Wireless sensor networks for personal health monitoring: issues and an implementation. Comput. Commun. **29**, 2521–2533 (2006)
3. Lin, J., Keogh, E., Lonardi, S., Chiu, B.: A symbolic representation of time series, with implications for streaming algorithms. In: 8th ACM SIGMOD Workshop on Research Issues in Data Mining and Knowledge Discovery, pp. 2–11, San Diego, CA (2003)
4. Shahar, Y.: A framework for knowledge-based temporal abstractions. Artif. Intell. **90**, 79–133 (1997)
5. Bellazzi, R., Larizza, C., Riva, A.: Temporal abstractions for interpreting diabetic patients monitoring data. Intell. Data Anal. **2**, 97–122 (1998)
6. Funk, P., Xiong, N.: Extracting knowledge from sensor signals for case-based reasoning with longitudinal time series data. In: Perner, P. (ed.) Case-Based Reasoning in Signals and Images, pp. 247–284. Springer, Heidelberg (2008)
7. Kullback, S., Leibler, R.A.: On information and sufficiency. Ann. Math. Stat. **22**, 79–86 (1951)
8. Massie, S., Wiratunga, N., Craw, S., Donati, A., Vicari, E.: From anomaly reports to cases. In: Weber, R.O., Richter, M.M. (eds.) ICCBR 2007. LNCS (LNAI), vol. 4626, pp. 359–373. Springer, Heidelberg (2007). doi:10.1007/978-3-540-74141-1_25
9. Mantaras, R.L.D., et al.: Retrieval, reuse, revision and retention in case-based reasoning. Knowl. Eng. Rev. **20**, 215–240 (2005)
10. Xiong, N.: A hybrid approach to input selection for complex processes. IEEE Trans. Sys. Man Cybern. Part A Syst. Hum. **32**, 532–536 (2002)
11. Xiong, N.: Fuzzy rule-based similarity model enables learning from small case bases. Appl. Soft Comput. **13**, 2057–2064 (2013)

A Classification Model for Predicting Heart Failure in Cardiac Patients

Muhammad Saqlain[(✉)], Rao Muzamal Liaqat, Nazar A. Saqib,
and Mazhar Hameed

College of Electrical and Mechanical Engineering (E&ME),
National University of Sciences and Technology (NUST), Islamabad, Pakistan
m.saqlain1240@yahoo.com, muzammilliaqat@gmail.com,
nazar.abbas@ce.ceme.edu.pk, mazharhameedsw@gmail.com

Abstract. Today the most significant public health problem is Heart Failure (HF). There are a lot of raw medical data available to healthcare organizations in the form of structured and unstructured datasets, but the need is to analyze this data to get information and to make intelligent decisions. By using data mining, classification tool on a real dataset of cardiac patients we propose a model which classified these patients into four major classes. This model will help to identify the risk of HF and patients who have no HF signs but structural irregularities. We can also identify the patients having HF signs and irregularities and those having the critical stage of HF. This paper provides a detailed summary of modern strategies for management and analysis of HF patients by classes (1 to 4) that have appeared in the past few years.

Keywords: Data mining · Classification techniques · Heart Failure · Predictive model · Support Vector Machine

1 Introduction

Heart failure (HF) has become a foremost reason for cardiovascular morbidity and mortality [1], and its occurrence is increasing day by day [2]. In common population, the chance of getting HF for a healthy person at 40 years of age is 1 in 5 [3]. It has become the key public health care precedence to control high HF patient's mortality rate [4]. It is the major goal for healthcare organizations to identify the cost-effective techniques to minimize the occurrence of hospitalization. An accurate prediction model can be very useful for physicians as well as for patients. Using this model a physician can recommend new insistent treatment plan and the patient can follow this plan more confidently [7].

Raw data collected from the patient's history can be very helpful for healthcare organizations if they can get the meaningful hidden patterns from it [5], and these hidden patterns are used to build predictive models for medical practitioners to control diseases and to making intelligent decisions before actual diseases occur. Data mining is one of the most important techniques for knowledge discovery in the dataset (KDD) and it can be used for disease prediction and for extracting hidden patterns [6]. There are a lot of databases available for healthcare organizations in the form of

© ICST Institute for Computer Sciences, Social Informatics and Telecommunications Engineering 2016
M.U. Ahmed et al. (Eds.): HealthyIoT 2016, LNICST 187, pp. 36–43, 2016.
DOI: 10.1007/978-3-319-51234-1_6

radiology reports, images, medication profiles, treatment records, signals, patient history, and pathology report. This type of data can be very complex, heterogeneous, noisy and uncertain [8].

In this research study, we take a real dataset of cardiac patient's by Armed Forces Institute of Cardiology (AFIC), Pakistan. We manually extract the important attribute of the unstructured dataset and propose a classification model using data mining, classification algorithms Support Vector Machine (SVM). We classify cardiac patients according to their conditions into four important classes as given below.

- Class 1: Patients with risk of HF
- Class 2: Patients having no HF symptoms, but structural heart irregularities
- Class 3: Patients having HF symptoms and structural heart irregularities
- Class 4: Patients with critical stage of HF

This study will present a detailed update on modern techniques in the management and diagnosis of heart failure by classes 1 to 4 that have to appear in the past few years. On behalf of various cardiac studies, we also present a treatment plan for patients belonging to different classes of our proposed model. This treatment plan will be very helpful for patients as well as for medical researchers and cardiologist to overcome the problem of each class separately. It will also focus on recent research results and strategies that may give the positive impact on clinical practice.

Section 2 contains the related research studies by different researchers of the same domain. In Sect. 3, we discuss our proposed classification model in detail. Section 4 contains the conclusion, which provides the overall summary of our research work.

2 Literature Review

Predictive modeling of cardiac disease using electronic health record (EHR) data has become a very broad research area. The reason behind this is that HF has become the main cause of death for adults [9]. There are many machine learning strategies available for classification, such as Logistic Regression (LR), Support Vector Machine (SVM), Random Forest (RF), Artificial Neural Network (ANN), Naïve Bayes (NB), Decision Trees (DT) and much more. In [10], the authors take data from the National Health and Nutrition Examination Survey (NHANES) and applied SVM for classification of diabetes patients and find Area under the Curve (AUC) of 83%. RF was applied by [11] for prediction the chances of depression due to Traumatic Brain Injury (TBI) identification. Authors of [12] take a dataset from EHR propose a model for detection of HF within the time period of 6 months before the real heart failure occurrence. They also provide the performance comparison of SVM, LR, and Boosting.

Data mining, classification strategies have being used for identification and prevention of cardiac diseases. In [13], the authors present a performance comparison on behalf of accuracy for ANN, SVM, DT, and RIPPER techniques. The results show that SVM with an accuracy of 84% was the best technique with all of these. An isolated cardiac detecting system was introduced for prevention of HF by [14], by using mobile gateways. This system extracted the highly related features and then applied SVM classifier and finds the accuracy of 87.5%. Authors of [15] take a real dataset from VA

Medical Center, California and provide the performance comparison of DT, ANN, and LR for prediction of cardiac disease and ANN show the highest accuracy. In [16] authors proposed a model to accept different strategies of machine learning to handle concealed dataset. They applied their model for predicting the repetition of cancer and give the performance comparison of DT, Cox regression, and NB. [17] Provided a prediction model to show HF patient's survival risk by using some common classification algorithms such as SVM, RF, DT, and LR. The results of their study show that LR provides the highest accuracy.

The authors of [21] present a classification system called Clinical Decision Support System (CDSS) for diagnosis purpose of cardiovascular disease by using four special classification methodologies (ANN, BN, SVM, and DT). Their system checks the disease level with an accuracy of more than 94%. An Intelligent Heart Disease Predication System (IHDPS) was presented by [22], used to extract hidden information and their relation with HF from a huge dataset of cardiac patients. This is a hybrid system created by three common data mining strategies: NB, DT, and ANN. They concluded that NB creates a more effective prediction. Another HF predictive system called "Intelligent and Effective Heart Attack Prediction System" (IEHAPS) was created by [23]. They use different methodologies of prediction: ANN, frequent pattern mining, and clustering. Maximum Frequent Itemset Algorithm (MAFIA) technique was used to filter most significant patterns and finally, ANN was trained by these patterns for prediction of heart failure in a very efficient manner.

3   HF Diagnosis and Prediction Model

There are many diseases and several other interrelated factors that may cause of HF for a normal person. That's why HF is a very heterogeneous disease and detection and prediction of this disease also a very tough job. So, data mining has introduced many algorithms that are being used to develop intelligent prediction models for physicians and medical practitioners which increase the accuracy of diagnosis of HF. In this study, we propose a data mining, classification model using real data of cardiac patients. Figure 1 shows the architectural view of our proposed model. We describe our model in different phases in detail as discussed below.

3.1   Data Preparation

We take raw data of 500 cardiac patients in the form of their medical reports from AFIC, Pakistan. We manually extract useful 32 features from these reports with the close collaboration of cardiologists and medical practitioners. We create a better understanding of these patient's medical reports with the help of cardiac specialists and make sure that these features are enough to get valuable results for our model. This approach provides a deep knowledge of cardiology and helps to understand the domain of the problem. These extracted features were stored in MS Excel to create a database. To make our data structured, we applied machine learning algorithms. Such as, we applied mapping table for transforming textual data into numeric data.

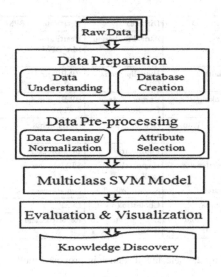

Fig. 1. Basic flow of proposed approach

3.2 Data Pre-processing

This phase includes several sub-processes such as data cleaning, data reduction, and data transformation. First, we handle identical, missing and inconsistent values in the dataset for cleaning purpose by removing and replacing with correct values. Finally, when we fed this dataset into database of Rapid Miner tool, it again cleans the dataset and replaced missing values with average value of that attribute by using an operator called "Replace Missing Value". "Normalize" operator was applied to cleaned dataset for standardization of data. This operator normalizes the attribute values of the selected attributes. Some important selected features are given in Fig. 2. By applying this strategy, we reduced the complexity of our dataset and it helps to develop a classification model with the highest accuracy [18].

3.3 Multi-class SVM Classification Modeling

Data was uploaded in Rapid Miner to develop SVM model. As SVM deal only with binary data, where our dataset contains multi-class data, so we applied "Class-Binarization" techniques to transform multi-class data into binary class data [19]. The dataset was managed into four subsets having individual class labels. Now we have four different classes' having the same number of attributes, but the diverse number of patients. SVM operator randomly takes 70% of the dataset for training. Now put the unseen 30% testing data into a trained model by "Apply Model" operator and find some valuable performance measures by applying "Performance" operator. It shows the results for each class and four separate models were created respectively. Our resulting attribute was "Result Class" and its categories are; Class 1, Class 2, Class 3 and Class 4.

Patient-ID	Diabetes	HeartRate-BI_BPM
Age	Atrial Fibrillation	HeartRate-MA_BPM
Gender	Hyperlipidemia	BP-BI_mmHg-uppLim
Smoking History	Chronic Kidney Disease	BP-BI_mmHg-lowLim
Family History	Ischemic Heart Disease	ACE inhibitor
BMI	Pulmonary	Beta-Blocker
Hypertension	Hemoglobin (g/dL)	STATIN user
Cataract	Sodium(mEq/L)	Diuretic user
Anemia	Cholestrol(mg/dL)	LVEF
Rheumatoid Arthritis	Lymphocytes(*10 (9)/L)	Reported Class

Fig. 2. Selected attributes in proposed model

3.4   Result Analysis

Different classification measures were used such as precision, classification error, sensitivity, specificity, F-measure, AUC, and accuracy to get the overall result of our model. Each class was evaluated individually and finally got overall results as shown in Table 1. All these resulting attributes are independent of each other, so higher the value of these attributes give the best performance of our prediction model. The result shows that a class having the highest value of accuracy will be the least value of precision and vice versa, as explained in [20]. By calculating the overall average result of all four classes we find the accuracy of the SVM model of 82%. As our dataset is very heterogeneous and have higher dimensional space, so we prefer SVM to other state-of-the-art classification models. SVM also gives better results for text classification.

Table 1. Accuracy measures for SVM models

SVM model	Precision (%)	F-Measure (%)	Sensitivity (%)	Classifi. error (%)	AUC (%)	Accuracy (%)
Class 1	81.97	88.5	96.15	8.67	96.8	91.33
Class 2	100	3.17	1.61	40.67	51.6	59.33
Class 3	100	8.7	4.55	14	73.8	86
Class 4	91.28	95.44	100	8.67	84.2	91.33
Average	93.3	68.53	50.58	18	76.6	81.99

3.5   Knowledge Discovery

On behalf of various cardiac studies and results of our model, we create an important treatment plan, explain in Fig. 3. Patients of class 1 are very common in our society because they ignore the risk of HF even they are already under attack of hypertension,

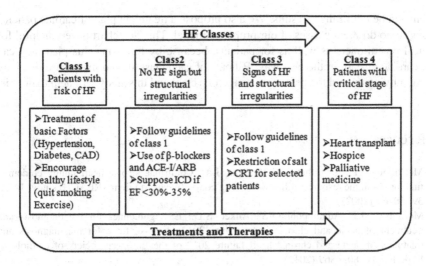

Fig. 3. Classes in development of HF and their suggested treatment

and diabetes. So patients with these diseases should never forget the risk of HF. They should promote their lifestyle to lose their weight and to quit smoking. Class 2 contains the patients that have some structural irregularities in the cardiac system and have more chances of HF, so they should be more careful about it. They should follow all instructions for class 1 patients and also should use β-blockers if they have reduced EF.

Patients of class 3 have symptoms of HF and they should prefer the use of diuretics. Patients of class 4 are in the most critical form of HF. These patients have preferred to use of palliative medicine or they are treated with heart transplants. So, this research study can be very helpful for cardiologists to treat the cardiac disease very efficiently.

Some important result of our study can be defined as:

- *Our dataset has 69% male patients, which conclude that the chances of HF are more in males than females.*
- *Dataset contains 73% of patients having more than 50 years of age, which means adults are more affected by this disease.*
- *We used SVM, a data mining algorithm to propose a classification model that classifies our data into 4 classes, which are very important for treatment of HF.*

4   Conclusion

This research study proposes a framework, in which we used a data set from AFIC, Pakistan. After applying all the necessary preprocessing steps of data mining we applied SVM, to classify our dataset into 4 important classes. Our proposed classification model gave the accuracy and AUC of 82% and 77% respectively. Our model with its excellent result is very helpful for medical practitioners to understand the causes of HF and they can make intelligent decisions to control the conditions of patients on behalf of these results. We also propose a treatment plan of cardiac patients belonging to different classes of our proposed model. This flowchart is very helpful for medical practitioners as well as for patients, because by following this plan they can treat cardiac disease in the best way. Patients of each class should make sure that they are not moving toward the next more dangerous class and this study will help to do this.

References

1. McCullough, P.A., Philbin, E.F., Spertus, J.A.: Confirmation of a heart failure epidemic: findings from the resource utilization among congestive heart failure (REACH) study. JACC **39**, 60–69 (2002)
2. McMurray, J.J., Adamopoulos, S., Anker, S.D.: ESC guidelines for the diagnosis and treatment of acute and chronic heart failure 2012: the task force for the diagnosis and treatment of acute and chronic heart failure 2012 of the European society of cardiology. EURJHF **14**, 803–869 (2012)
3. Ouwerkerk, W., Adriaan, A.V., Zwinderman, A.H.: Factors influencing the predictive power of models for predicting mortality and/or heart failure hospitalization in patients with heart failure. JACC. Heart Fail **2**, 429–436 (2014)
4. Gerber, Y., Weston, S.A., Redfiled, M.M., Chamberlain, A.M., Manemann, S.M., Killian, J. M., Roger, V.L.: A contemporary appraisal of the heart failure epidemic in Olmsted county, Minnesota, 2000 to 2010. JAMA Intern. Med. **175**, 996 (2015)
5. Tan, G., Cbye, H.: Data mining applications in healthcare. J. Healthcare Inf. Manage. **19**, 64 (2004)
6. Giudici, P.: Applied Data Mining: Statistical Methods for Business and Industry. Wiley, New York (2003)
7. Taslimitehrani, V., Dong, G.: Developing EHR-driven heart failure risk prediction models using CPXR (Log) with the probabilistic loss function. J. Biomed. Inform. **60**, 260–269 (2016)
8. Cios, K.J., Moore, G.W.: Uniqueness of medical data mining. Intell Med. **26**, 1–24 (2002)
9. Health World Organization: The top 10 causes of death. http://www.who.int/mediacentre/factsheets/fs310/en/index.html
10. Wei, Y., Liu, T., Valdez, R., Gwinn, M., Khoury, M.J.: Application of support vector machine modeling for prediction of common diseases: the case of diabetes and pre-diabetes. BMC Med. Inform. Decis. Mak. **10**, 16 (2010)
11. Kennedy, R.E., Livingston, L., Riddick, A., Marwitz, J.H., Kreutzer, J.S., Zasler, N.D.: Evaluation of the neurobehavioral functioning inventory as a depression screening tool after traumatic brain injury. Jorn. Head Trauma Rehab. **20**, 512–526 (2005)
12. Wu, J., Roy, J., Stewart, W.F.: Prediction modeling using EHR data: challenges, strategies, and a comparison of machine learning approaches. Med. Care **48**, 106–113 (2010)
13. Kumari, M., Godara, S.: Comparative study of data mining classification methods in cardiovascular disease prediction. IJCST **2** (2009)
14. Kwon, K., Hwang, H., Kang, H., Woo, K.G., Shim, K.: A remote cardiac monitoring system for preventive care. In: Proceedings of ICCE, pp. 197–200. IEEE (2013)
15. Kurt, I., Ture, M., Kurum, A.T.: Comparing performances of logistic regression, classification and regression tree, and neural networks for predicting coronary artery disease. Expert Syst. Appl. **34**, 366–374 (2008)

16. Zupan, B., Demsar, J., Kattan, M.W., Beck, J.R., Bratko, I.: Machine learning for survival analysis: a case study on recurrence of prostate cancer. Artif. Intell. Med. **20**, 59–75 (2000)
17. Panahiazar, M., Taslimitehrani, V., Pereira, N., Pathak, J.: Using EHRs and machine learning for heart failure survival analysis. Study Health Technol. Inform. Med. **216**, 40–44 (2015)
18. Deekshatulu, B.L., Chandra, P.: Classification of heart disease using artificial neural network and feature subset selection. Global J. Comput. Sci. Technol. **13** (2013)
19. Fürnkranz, J.: Round Robin classification. J. Mac. Learn. Res. **2**, 721–747 (2002)
20. http://www.ncsu.edu/labwrite/Experimental%20Design/accuracyprecision.htm
21. Hong, J., Kim, S., Zhang, B.: AptaCDSS-E: a classifier ensemble-based clinical decision support system for cardiovascular disease level prediction. Expert Syst. Appl. **34**, 2465 (2008)
22. Awang, R., Palaniappan, S.: Intelligent heart disease predication system using data mining technique. Int. J. Comput. Sci. Netw. Secur. **8** (2008)
23. Patil, S., Kumaraswamy, Y.: Intelligent and effective heart attack prediction system using data mining and artificial neural network. Eur. J. Sci. Res. **31** (2009)

Ins and Outs of Big Data: A Review

Hamidur Rahman$^{(\boxtimes)}$, Shahina Begum, and Mobyen Uddin Ahmed

School of Innovation, Design and Engineering,
Mälardalens University, Västerås, Sweden
{hamidur.rahman,shahina.begum,
mobyenuddin.ahmed}@mdh.se

Abstract. Today with the fast development of digital technologies and advance communications a gigantic amount of data sets with massive and complex structures called 'Big data' is being produced everyday enormously and exponentially. Again, the arrival of social media, advent of smart homes, offices and hospitals are connected as Internet of Things (IoT), this influence also a lot to Big data. According to the study, Big data presents data sets with large magnitude including structured, semi-structured or unstructured data. The study also presents the new technologies for data analyzing, collecting, fast searching, proper sharing, exact storing, speedy transferring, hidden pattern visualization and violations of privacy etc. This paper presents an overview of ins and outs of Big Data where the content, scope, samples, methods, advantages, challenges and privacy of Big data have been discussed. The goal of this article is to provide big data knowledge to the research community for the sake of its many real life applications such as traffic management, driver monitoring, health care in hospitals, meteorology and so on.

Keywords: Big data issue · Framework · Analytics · Challenges · Tools

1 Introduction

The 'Big data' term has come into the research community more clearly during 2013 and afterwards. Several authors have tried to explain the definition and the possible issues, technologies, challenges and privacy of big data in a concise way [1–5]. For example in 2001, Laney et al. have highlighted the challenges and opportunities generated by increased data through a 3Vs model, i.e., increases in volume, velocity and variety [6]. In recent years, the world has become so much digitalized and interconnected and as a result the amount of data has been exploding. Therefore, to manage the massive amount of records it requires extremely powerful business intelligence. The problem may arise even more during data acquisition if the amount of data is too large and then it may have a confusion level that what data to keep and what to discard and how to store the data in a reliable way. A clear definition of Big data has been using for the accumulation of different sort of huge amount of data since last 2–3 years. In 2015, the digital world expanded to 5.6 exabytes (10^{18} bytes) of data created each day. This figure is expected to double by every 24 months or so [7]. As a result, storing, managing, sharing, analyzing and visualizing information via typical database software tools is not only so difficult but also very hazardous task. Big data can be structured,

© ICST Institute for Computer Sciences, Social Informatics and Telecommunications Engineering 2016
M.U. Ahmed et al. (Eds.): HealthyIoT 2016, LNICST 187, pp. 44–51, 2016.
DOI: 10.1007/978-3-319-51234-1_7

semi-structured and unstructured in nature but it could help in businesses by producing automated services to target their potential partners, agents or customers.

There are some Big data review articles available in online but most of them have emphasized on specific area e.g., big data framework, big challenges, big data applications etc. but almost all of them have failed to provide complete overview of Big data [2, 8, 9]. In this paper, we have presented a complete overview of Big Data and its present state-of-the-art. Additionally, we have tried to find out big data important characteristics, Big data frameworks and analytic, challenges of big data and possible solutions, big data tools and its applications in famous companies. This article will be very helpful for new researchers specially data scientist, research institutes and companies to get insights view and latest technologies of big data for their research planning, business activities and future demand for handling massive amount of data.

2 Materials and Methods

The Big data is relatively a new topic and the amount of research articles published so far is limited in this area. Around 60 Big data related articles have been collected from different online sources where IEEE explore, Research Gate and Google Scholar databases are the privileged sources. Some of the articles were searched using google Chrome search engine and during the searching period different key words were used such as 'big data', 'big data issues', 'big data challenges', 'big data analytics', 'recent trend of big data' etc. and it was also considered the most recent articles which are available in online database. In our case we only considered the articles published in between 2013 to 2016. About 70% of the collected articles were considered for detailed study through the paper and remaining 30% of the articles are excluded due to similarity with considered articles and less important for the study.

3 Big Data Characteristics

Big data is usually characterized by the three dimensions or 3 V called Volume, Velocity and Variety [6]. However, other dimensions presented in Fig. 1 such as variety, validity and value can be at least equally important. According to the study, additional three dimensions Veracity, Validity and Value have considered and presented in Fig. 1 with "6 Vs" of big data. The 1st V is Volume which concerns the fact of amount of generated data that is increasing tremendously in each day. The second V is Velocity which has come into light due to more and more data and is provided to the users immediately whenever required for real time processing. Variety is the 3rd V considered due to the tremendous growth in data sources which are needed for analysis.

Veracity which includes trust in the information received, is often cited as an important 4th V dimension in addition to big Data. Validity does not only involve ensuring accurate measurements but also the transparency of assumptions and connections behind the process. Value refers to recent large volumes of data measured in exabytes, petabytes or higher ranked of data and highly valuable for research institutes and industries.

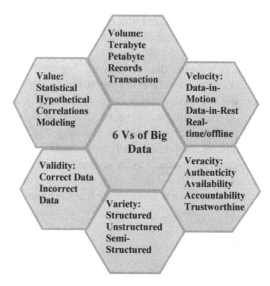

Fig. 1. The important characteristics of Big data (6 V's)

4   Big Data Analytic and Frameworks

In general view, data analytics is one of the major part in Big data environment which is responsible to simplify complexity of the data and calculation for achieving of expected pattern of data sets and outcome. As a whole, there are 3 main tasks in Big data framework which includes initial planning, implementation and evaluation and all the tasks have 8 layers as described in Fig. 2 [1].

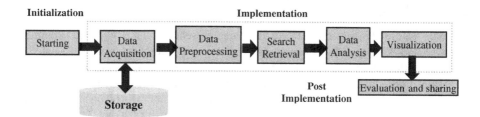

Fig. 2. Layers of big data analytic task and framework

Initialization: The first layer of any Big data framework is the primary planning which requires new investments for big changes and the changes basically include installation of a new technological infrastructure and a new way to process and control data [10]. At the beginning it is extremely important to find problems that needs a solution and decision whether they could be solved using new technologies or just with available software and techniques. These problems could be large volume challenges, real time processing, predictive analytics, on-demand analytics and so on.

Implementation: The second task is implementation and there are several activities such as data storage, pre-processing, search retrieval, analysis and visualization. To overcome the storage capacity problem cloud computing technology has a great advantage [11, 12] and provides easy access for applications from different corners of the world. Data analysis is one of the most important steps in implementation where various preprocessing operations are necessary to address different imperfections in collected raw data. As the data sources are different multi-source data fusion technology such as [13–15] could be applied. After that all the data must be pre-processed to avoid similarity, remove noise and delete unwanted signals [16–20]. For example, data can have multiple formats as heterogeneous sources are involved. It can also mix with noises where unnecessary data, errors, outliers etc. are included. Additionally, it may subsequently necessary to fit requirements of analysis algorithms. Therefore, data preprocessing includes a wide range of operations such as cleaning, integration, reduction, normalization, transformation, discretization etc.

When the pre-processing stage is done then the search retrieval is performed to extract values for further analysis for companies and institutions. Advance analytics is one of the most efficient approaches which provides algorithms such as descriptive analytics, inquisitive analytics, predictive and prescriptive analytics to perform complex analytics on either structured or unstructured data. When the analyzing part is done then the visualization is very important where it guides the analysis process and presents the summary of the results in a transparent, understandable and meaningful way. For the simple graphical representation of data, most software packages support classical charts and dashboards.

Evaluation and Sharing: The third task of the big data framework is evaluation the outcome and sharing it among the agents [10]. To evaluate a Big data project, it is necessary to consider a range of diverse data inputs, quality of data and expected results. To develop procedures for Big Data evaluation, the project first needs to allow real time stream processing and incremental computation of statistics. There is also necessity to have parallel processing and exploitation of distributed computing so that data can be processed in a reasonable amount of time. It is also considering that the project can easily be integrated with visualization tools. Finally, it should perform summary indexing to accelerate queries on big datasets to accelerate running queries.

5 Big Data Challenges and Inconsistencies

Context awareness is one of the major analytic challenge that focuses on some portions of data and which is useful for resource consumption [3]. Another crucial challenge is visual analysis that how data seems to be for the perception of human vision. Similarly, data efficiency, correlation between the features of data and contents validation are notable challenges. Data privacy, security and trust are also major concern among organizations. When volume of data grows, it is difficult to gain insight into data within time period. Processing near real time data will always require processing interval in order to produce satisfactory output. Transition between structured data- stored in well-defined tables and unstructured data (images, videos, text) required for analysis will affect end to end processing of data. Invention of new non-relational technologies will provide some flexibility in data representation and processing.

In circumstances where big data are collected, aggregated, transformed or represented inconsistencies invariably find their way into large datasets [21]. This can be attributed to a number of factors in human behaviors and in decision-making process. When datasets contain a temporal attribute, data items with conflicting circumstances may coincide or overlap in time. The time interval relationships between conflicting data items can result in partial temporal inconsistency. Spatial inconsistencies can be arisen from the geometric representation of objects, spatial relations between objects or aggregation of composite objects. As big datasets are increasingly generated from social media, blogs, emails, crowd-sourced ratings, inconsistencies in unstructured text and messages become an important research topic. If two texts are referring to the same event or entity, then they are said to be of co-reference. Event or entity co-referencing is a necessary condition for text inconsistencies.

6 Big Data Domain, Technology, Tools and Solution

Big Data domain has no boundary including retail application to governmental works. A big data might be petabyte (1024 terabyte) or Exabyte (1024 petabyte) of data consisting of billions to trillions of records of millions of people from different sources like educational institutions, research institutions, medical hospitals, small or multi-national company data, customer care, weather records, demographical data, social media records, astronomical data etc. [21]. These massive data sets and its applications include technologies such Mathematics, Artificial Intelligence Especially Machine Learning, Data Mining, Cloud Computing, Real Time Data Streaming technology and so on [21]. Time series analysis is also very useful and of course there are many visualization technologies that can be used in Big data.

Today most of the renowned companies are using big data tools for their special needs. For example, Hadoop[1] and MongoDB[2] are the two best data storage and management tool used by Google, Amazon and MIT, MTV respectively. For data cleaning, Stratebi and Platon companies are using DataCleaner[3] tool. Teradata[4] is another big data tool for data mining used by Air Canada or cisco. Autodesk company uses Qubole[5] for their data analysis. For big data visualization, Plot.ly[6] is one of the greatest and many renowned companies like Google, Goji, VTT are using this tool. For the data integration, Pentaho[7] is one of the best tool used by CAT, Logitech etc.

---

[1] http://wiki.apache.org/hadoop/PoweredBy#G.

[2] https://www.mongodb.com/industries.

[3] https://datacleaner.org/testimonials.

[4] http://www.teradata.se/customers-list/browse/?LangType=1053&LangSelect=true.

[5] https://www.qubole.com/customer/?nabe=5695374637924352:1.

[6] https://plot.ly/#trusted-by.

[7] http://www.pentaho.com/customers.

Table 1. Big data tools used by renowned companies

No	Big data tools	Where it is used
1	Hadoop	Google, Amazon, Alibaba, Facebook etc.
2	MongoDB	citiGroup, MIT, GOV.UK, ebay, MTV etc.
3	DataCleaner	Stratebi, Platon, BestBrains etc.
4	Teradata	Air Canada, cisco, Coca-Cola, Coop, Dell, Daimler etc.
5	Qubole	Autodesk, Answers.com, Capilary, Quora, Nextdoor, etc.
6	Plot.ly	Google, Goji, VTT, U.S. Air Force etc.
7	Pentaho	CAT, Nasdaq, Logitech, U.S. Navy etc.
8	Python	Forecastwatch.com, AstraZeneca, Carmanah etc.
9	Import.io	Quid, Nygg, OpenRise, University of Houston etc.

Python[8] is widely used as a Big data language for company like AstraZeneca, Carmanah etc. As a big data collection tool Import.io[9] is pioneer and used by Quid, Nygg, OpenRise etc. A list of Big data tools used by famous companies are listed in Table 1.

There are thousands of Big data tools both available in the market to buy and also for free trial for extraction, storage, cleaning, mining, visualizing, analyzing and integrating. Table 2 shows the most popular big data tools.

Table 2. A number of popular big data tools (https://www.import.io/post/all-the-best-big-data-tools-and-how-to-use-them/).

No	Big data area	Tools
1	Data Storage and Management	Hadoop, Cloudera, MongoDB, Talend
2	Data Cleaning	OpenRefine, DataCleaner
3	Data Mining	RapidMiner, Teradata, FramedData, Kaggle
4	Data Analysis	Qubole, BigML, Statwing
5	Data Visualization	Tableau, Silk, CartoDB, Chartio, Plot.ly,
6	Data Integration	Blockspring, Pentaho
7	Data Languages	R, Python, RegEx, XPath
8	Data Collection	Import.io

7 Conclusion

A general overview and concept of the Big data has been discussed in this article including Big data 6 V, it's framework and analytic issues. Additionally, the difference between big and small data, popular tools, inconsistencies and challenges also have been reviewed. Due to management and analysis of petabytes and exabytes of data, the big data management system cooperates and ensures a high level of data quality, accessibility and helps to locate valuable information in large set of unstructured and

---

[8] https://www.python.org/about/success/#engineering.
[9] https://www.import.io/.

unplanned data. This review of different techniques can be applied to various fields of engineering, industry and medical science. Some real life applications such as autonomous driving, smooth transaction for semi-autonomous driving or driver monitoring in context of big data analysis will be presented as future work.

Acknowledgement. The authors would like to acknowledge the Swedish Knowledge Foundation (KKS), Swedish Governmental agency for innovation Systems (VINNOVA), Volvo Car Corporation, The Swedish National Road and Transportation Research Institute, Autoliv AB, Hök instrument AB, and Prevas AB Sweden for their support of the research projects in this area.

References

1. Tekiner, F., Keane, J.A.: Big data framework. In: 2013 IEEE International Conference on Systems, Man, and Cybernetics, pp. 1494–1499 (2013)
2. Sagiroglu, S., Sinanc, D.: Big data: a review. In: 2013 International Conference on Collaboration Technologies and Systems (CTS), pp. 42–47 (2013)
3. Katal, A., Wazid, M., Goudar, R.H.: Big data: issues, challenges, tools and good practices. In: 2013 Sixth International Conference on Contemporary Computing (IC3), pp. 404–409 (2013)
4. Xiong, W., Yu, Z., Bei, Z., Zhao, J., Zhang, F., Zou, Y., et al.: A characterization of big data benchmarks. In: 2013 IEEE International Conference on Big Data, pp. 118–125 (2013)
5. Lu, T., Guo, X., Xu, B., Zhao, L., Peng, Y., Yang, H.: Next big thing in big data: the security of the ICT supply chain. In: 2013 International Conference on Social Computing (SocialCom), pp. 1066–1073 (2013)
6. Laney, D.: 3-D data management: controlling data volume, velocity and variety. META Group Original Research Note (2001)
7. Ahmed, F.D., Jaber, A.N., Majid, M.B.A., Ahmad, M.S.: Agent-based big data analytics in retailing: a case study. In: 2015 4th International Conference on Software Engineering and Computer Systems (ICSECS), pp. 67–72 (2015)
8. Gupta, P., Tyagi, N.: An approach towards big data-a review. In: 2015 International Conference on Computing, Communication & Automation (ICCCA), pp. 118–123 (2015)
9. Rout, T., Garanayak, M., Senapati, M.R., Kamilla, S.K.: Big data and its applications: a review. In: 2015 International Conference on Electrical, Electronics, Signals, Communication and Optimization (EESCO), pp. 1–5 (2015)
10. Mousannif, H., Sabah, H., Douiji, Y., Sayad, Y.O.: From big data to big projects: a step-by-step roadmap. In: 2014 International Conference on Future Internet of Things and Cloud (FiCloud), pp. 373–378 (2014)
11. Huang, G., He, J., Chi, C.H., Zhou, W., Zhang, Y.: A data as a product model for future consumption of big stream data in clouds. In: 2015 IEEE International Conference on Services Computing (SCC), pp. 256–263 (2015)
12. Khan, I., Naqvi, S.K., Alam, M., Rizvi, S.N.A.: Data model for big data in cloud environment. In: 2015 2nd International Conference on Computing for Sustainable Global Development (INDIACom), pp. 582–585 (2015)
13. Suciu, G., Vulpe, A., Craciunescu, R., Butca, C., Suciu, V.: Big data fusion for eHealth and ambient assisted living cloud applications. In: 2015 IEEE International Black Sea Conference on Communications and Networking (BlackSeaCom), pp. 102–106 (2015)

14. Yang, L.T., Kuang, L., Chen, J., Hao, F., Luo, C.: A holistic approach to distributed dimensionality reduction of big data. IEEE Trans. Cloud Comput. **PP**, 1 (2015)
15. Zheng, Y.: Methodologies for cross-domain data fusion: an overview. IEEE Trans. Big Data **1**, 16–34 (2015)
16. Pandey, S., Tokekar, V.: Prominence of MapReduce in big data processing. In: 2014 Fourth International Conference on Communication Systems and Network Technologies (CSNT), pp. 555–560 (2014)
17. Wang, J., Song, Z., Li, Q., Yu, J., Chen, F.: Semantic-based intelligent data clean framework for big data. In: 2014 International Conference on Security, Pattern Analysis, and Cybernetics (SPAC), pp. 448–453 (2014)
18. Biookaghazadeh, S., Xu, Y., Zhou, S., Zhao, M.: Enabling scientific data storage and processing on big-data systems. In: 2015 IEEE International Conference on Big Data (Big Data), pp. 1978–1984 (2015)
19. Diao, Y., Liu, K.Y., Meng, X., Ye, X., He, K.: A big data online cleaning algorithm based on dynamic outlier detection. In: 2015 International Conference on Cyber-Enabled Distributed Computing and Knowledge Discovery (CyberC), pp. 230–234 (2015)
20. Taleb, I., Dssouli, R., Serhani, M.A.: Big data pre-processing: a quality framework. In: 2015 IEEE International Congress on Big Data, pp. 191–198 (2015)
21. Zhang, D.: Inconsistencies in big data. In: 2013 12th IEEE International Conference on Cognitive Informatics & Cognitive Computing (ICCI*CC), pp. 61–67 (2013)

A Review of Parkinson's Disease Cardinal and Dyskinetic Motor Symptoms Assessment Methods Using Sensor Systems

Somayeh Aghanavesi[(✉)] and Jerker Westin

Computer Science Department, Dalarna University,
Rodavagen 3, S78188 Borlänge, Sweden
{saa,jwe}@du.se

Abstract. This paper is reviewing objective assessments of Parkinson's disease (PD) motor symptoms, cardinal, and dyskinesia, using sensor systems. It surveys the manifestation of PD symptoms, sensors that were used for their detection, types of signals (measures) as well as their signal processing (data analysis) methods. A summary of this review's finding is represented in a table including devices (sensors), measures and methods that were used in each reviewed motor symptom assessment study. In the gathered studies among sensors, accelerometers and touch screen devices are the most widely used to detect PD symptoms and among symptoms, bradykinesia and tremor were found to be mostly evaluated. In general, machine learning methods are potentially promising for this. PD is a complex disease that requires continuous monitoring and multidimensional symptom analysis. Combining existing technologies to develop new sensor platforms may assist in assessing the overall symptom profile more accurately to develop useful tools towards supporting better treatment process.

Keywords: Parkinson's Disease · Sensors · Objective assessment · Motor symptoms · Machine learning · Dyskinesia · Bradykinesia · Rigidity · Tremor

1 Introduction

The number of studies using electronic healthcare technologies and sensor systems assessing the Parkinson's disease (PD) motor symptoms objectively are increasing. PD is a progressive neurological disorder characterized by a large number of motor symptoms that can impact on the function to a variable degree. The four cardinal motor symptoms of PD comprise of tremor, rigidity, bradykinesia and postural instability. The primary goal of therapy is to maintain good motor function. Therefore therapeutic decision making requires accurate, comprehensive and accessible quantification of symptoms. Electronic sensor-based systems can facilitate remote, long-term and repeated symptom assessments. They are able to capture the symptom fluctuations more accurately and also they are effective with patient's hospitalization costs. This paper reviews methods and sensor systems to detect, assess and quantify the four cardinal and dyskinetic motor symptoms. The method for identifying and accessing resources involved the online databases, Google Scholar, IEEE computer society,

© ICST Institute for Computer Sciences, Social Informatics and Telecommunications Engineering 2016
M.U. Ahmed et al. (Eds.): HealthyIoT 2016, LNICST 187, pp. 52–57, 2016.
DOI: 10.1007/978-3-319-51234-1_8

Springer link (Springer Netherlands) and PubMed central. The evaluation of resources was based on their relevance to the topic and the year of publication (not older than 2005). Selection of articles is done to have one reference per instrument that was used to detect all our addressed symptoms. The structure of this article is formed into sections of PD symptoms, followed by corresponding sensors and instruments, and computer and statistical methods that were employed for assessments.

2 Parkinson's Disease Cardinal and Dyskinetic Symptoms

Parkinson's tremor consists of oscillating movements and appears when a person's muscles are relaxed and disappears when the person starts an action. It's the most apparent well-known symptom. Rigidity symptoms cause stiffness of the limbs, neck or trunk and result in inflexibility. Bradykinesia (slow movement) describes the general reduction of spontaneous movement (abnormal stillness and a decrease in facial expressivity) and causes difficulties with repetitive movements. It can cause walking with short and shuffling steps and can also affect the speech. Postural instability symptom is a trend to be unstable when standing upright, rising from a chair or turning. And dyskinesia is a difficulty in performing voluntary movements, which often occurs as a side effect of long-term therapy with levodopa. Dyskinetic movements look like smooth tics (uncoordinated periodic moves).

3 Sensors, Signals and Measures

Among the developed electronic techniques to measure and analyze the PD's symptoms the common sensors and devices for evaluation are accelerometer, electromyograph (EMG), magnetic tracker system, gyroscope, digitizing tablet, video recording, motion detector, and depth sensor. In accelerometry, an electromechanical sensor device is used to measure acceleration forces and capture the movements by converting it into electrical signals that are proportional to the muscular force producing motion. Gyroscope is a sensor device used to measure angular velocity (angular rate) which senses rotational motion and changes in orientation [1]. Accelerometer and gyroscope are joint in many motion sensing instruments. Electromyography (EMG) is a technique for evaluating and recording the electrical activity produced by neurologically activated muscles using Electromyograph that records how fast nerves can send electrical signals. Digitizing tablet in PD symptom detection is a computer input device used to digitize patient's drawing when he/she traces a pre-drawn shape [2] or freely writes or draws a shape. The position of the tip of the pen (x, y) and the time (milliseconds) are collected for analysis [3]. Electromagnetic tracker system captures the object's movement displacement (x, y, and z) and orientation (pitch, roll, and yaw). Active optical marker systems are used to capture and record object's motion. Wired position markers can be placed on different locations of patient's body to obtain object's posture and movements.

4 Signal Processing and Analysis

Wavelet transform as a multi-resolution transformation method uses a variable window size at each level to obtain more information about the sensor signal in the time-frequency (time-scale) domain. Principal component analysis (PCA) is theoretically the best linear dimension reduction technique that uses rectangular transformation to convert the set of observations of possibly correlated variables into a set of values of linearly uncorrelated variables [3]. It's the direction to where the most variance exists. Wavelet transform is usually used with PCA to reduce the number of features to most important and related ones [3]. Discrete Fourier Transform converts samples of a function (a signal that varies over time) into the list of coefficients of a finite combination of complex sinusoids (ordered frequency that has sample value). Fast Fourier transform converts time (signal) to frequency by decomposing an N point time domain signal into N signals [4] and Detrended Fluctuation Analysis is a method to determine self-affection of a signal [5]. Often Spectral Analysis (SA) is used in signal processing for PD's motor symptom assessment. The magnitude of an input signal versus a certain frequency within the full range of the frequency is measured using a spectrum analyzer. Artificial Intelligence (Visual perception, decision making, image processing, and classification techniques) enables the development of computer systems to perform tasks that usually require human intelligence. For image processing, computer vision is a method to acquire, process and analyze a patient body's images (like face and body posture). Machine learning in PD symptom assessment [6] often includes techniques to assess the magnitude of addressed symptom. Linear discriminant analysis (LDA) classification method is used to optimally separate populations and reduce the dimensionality [7]. Non-parametric, generalized and multilayer perceptron analysis are different alternatives of LDA.

5 Discussion and Conclusion

Table 1 summarizes the research studies that have evaluated the four cardinal PD motor symptoms. From left to right, it lists the evaluated symptoms, type of the instruments, calculated measures and employed analytical assessment methods.

Table 1. An overview of research studies articles that objectively assess PD motor symptoms and dyskinesia (Spectral Analysis is abbreviated as SA, and three dimension as 3-D).

Symptom	Instrument	Measure	Method	Reference
Tremor	Smartphone (3-D accelerometer, timer, finger tappning sensor)	X and Y coordinates, Time duration, 3-D Acceleration	Random forest machine learning technique, Detrended analysis	[5], 2015
	Pen stylus	Acceleration	Non parametric	[9], 2013
Rigidity	Real time wearable sensor	Acceleration	Shank, Ankle, Knee signal SA	[10], 2010

(continued)

Table 1. (*continued*)

Symptom	Instrument	Measure	Method	Reference
	Custom made goniometer	Angular velocity	SA of vertical leg acceleration	[11], 2010
	Stride monitor system	Acceleration	Extension-flexion-component analysis	[12], 2008
	Isokinetic dynamometer Biodex System 3	3-D angular velocity, Anatomical zero	Spearman correlation	[13], 2014
Dyskinesia	Digitized tablet (Spirography)	Velocity of drawing movements	Standard deviation analysis of drawing velocity	[2], 2005
	Wrist accelerometer	Trunk acceleration, Shank velocity	Support vector Machine learning	[6], 2012
	Wrist-worn inertial sensor	Median angular velocity of trunk Rotation	Linear discriminant analysis	[7], 2015
Postural instability	MTX Xsens sensor with 3-D accelerometer and 3-D gyroscope	Acceleration, Direction and Distance	Antero-posterior (AP), Medio-lateral (ML), and Vertical directions analysis	[14], 2011
	Motion detector, Depth sensor, Vicon, motion capture system and Force plate	Ground reaction force, Body center of mass, Displacement, Velocity	Segmental method, Zero-point-to-zero-point integration technique	[15], 2014
	Digital angular-velocity transducer	Velocity (pitch, roll, angle), Time	Linear discriminant analysis, Anova	[8], 2005
	Accelerometer	Acceleration	Posture contextualization algorithm	[16], 2014
Tremor and Dyskinesia	Accelerometer, Gyroscope, Infrared camera	Acceleration, Angular velocity and time	Genetic Algorithm spectral classification	[20], 2014
Tremor and Bradykinesia	Miniature uni-axial gyroscope	Angular velocity in roll, yaw and pitch direction	Biomedical signal processing (Spectrum Analysis)	[1], 2007
Tremor and Postural instability	Accelerometer	Mean velocity, Acceleration range, Mean acceleration	Hilbert–Huang transformation of postural parameters	[17], 2011
Bradykinesia and Dyskinesia	Digitized tablet (spiral and tapping) Pocket PC device	Radius, Time, Mean speed of correct proportion of taps	Wavelet transform and principal component analysis	[3], 2010
	Ambulatory Multichannel accelerometer, Video recorder	Acceleration, Body position, Time, Gravitational force, Body segment angel	Direct current component, Discriminant, variance (Anova), regression analysis	[18], 2005
	Kinetigraph(3-D accelerometer)	Time period, Wrist acceleration	Expert system approach	[19], 2012
Rigidity, Bradykinesia and Dyskinesia	Digitized tablet with finger tapping and Spirography	Speed, Accuracy, Standard deviation of radial drawing velocity	Principal component analysis	[4], 2010

According to Table 1, rigidity and postural instability are mostly evaluated as single symptoms. However, among articles which research on combined symptoms assessments, bradykinesia (with tremor, dyskinesia, rigidity, and dyskinesia together) is mostly studied. Tremor is assessed in some studies as a single symptom, and also together with each of bradykinesia, dyskinesia, and postural instability symptoms.

A common sensor for symptom detection was the accelerometer that was mostly used for detecting the tremor, dyskinesia, and postural instability. Digitizing tablet is used almost for all types of symptoms. Smartphone [5] and Microsoft Kinect (motion detector, and depth sensor) [15] are the latest devices in the market used for this. Smartphones (new generation of sensing devices) could expand rapidly with PD motor symptom assessments. Angular sensor detectors are used to detect rigidity and postural instability as single symptoms, and they are also used to detect bradykinesia and dyskinesia together with tremor. Video recording is often required for clinicians' observational analysis. Wearable sensors (small, available, accurate, including high time resolution, and flexible with body locations) are preferred for PD since it's a progressive chronic disease and symptoms need to be assessed continuously throughout the day. For this, the mobile applications and wrist watches are more preferred as they are currently part of almost everyone's daily accessories. However, their analysis methods and their validations are important and a question is whether the devices or clinical ratings will become the gold standard. Machine learning techniques are potentially good solutions in the development of assessment systems to determine the effectiveness of drug dosing. Tools that can effectively characterize the severity of symptoms and can discriminate between bradykinesia and dyskinesia are needed. Some successful products are Parkinson's Kinetigraph [18], Kinesia devices [20], and Rempark [6].

References

1. Salarian, A., et al.: Quantification of tremor and bradykinesia in Parkinson's disease using a novel ambulatory monitoring system. IEEE Trans. Biomed. Eng. **54**(2), 313–322 (2007)
2. Liu, X., et al.: Quantifying drug-induced dyskinesias in the arms using digitised spiral-drawing tasks. J. Neurosci. Meth. **144**(1), 47–52 (2005)
3. Westin, J., et al.: A new computer method for assessing drawing impairment in Parkinson's disease. J. Neurosci. Meth. **190**(1), 143–148 (2010)
4. Westin, J., et al.: A home environment test battery for status assessment in patients with advanced Parkinson's disease. Comput. Meth. Programs Biomed. **98**(1), 27–35 (2010)
5. Arora, S., et al.: Detecting and monitoring the symptoms of Parkinson's disease using smartphones: a pilot study. Parkinsonism Relat. Dis. **21**(6), 650–653 (2015)
6. Sama, A., et al.: Dyskinesia and motor state detection in Parkinson's disease patients with a single movement sensor. Conf. Proc. IEEE Eng. Med. Biol. Soc. **2012**, 1194–1197 (2012)
7. Lopane, G., et al.: Dyskinesia detection and monitoring by a single sensor in patients with Parkinson's disease. Mov. Disord. **30**, 1267 (2015)
8. Adkin, A.L., Bloem, B.R., Allum, J.H.J.: Trunk sway measurements during stance and gait tasks in Parkinson's disease. Gait Posture **22**(3), 240–249 (2005)

9. Scanlon, B.K., et al.: An accelerometry-based study of lower and upper limb tremor in Parkinson's disease. J. Clin. Neurosci. **20**(6), 827–830 (2013)
10. Bachlin, M., et al.: A wearable system to assist walking of Parkinson s disease patients. Meth. Inf. Med. **49**(1), 88–95 (2010)
11. Moreau, C., et al.: Gait disorders in Parkinson's disease: and pathophysiological approaches. Rev. Neurol. (Paris) **166**(2), 158–167 (2010)
12. Moore, S.T., MacDougall, H.G., Ondo, W.G.: Ambulatory monitoring of freezing of gait in Parkinson's disease. J. Neurosci. Meth. **167**(2), 340–348 (2008)
13. Cano-de-la-Cuerda, R., et al.: Isokinetic dynamometry as a technologic assessment tool for trunk rigidity in Parkinson's disease patients. NeuroRehabilitation **35**(3), 493–501 (2014)
14. Mancini, M., et al.: Trunk accelerometry reveals postural instability in untreated Parkinson's disease. Parkinsonism Relat. Disord. **17**(7), 557–562 (2011)
15. Yeung, L.F., et al.: Evaluation of the Microsoft Kinect as a clinical assessment tool of body sway. Gait Posture **40**(4), 532–538 (2014)
16. Ahlrichs, C., et al.: Detecting freezing of gait with a tri-axial accelerometer in Parkinson's disease patients. Med. Biol. Eng. Comput. **54**(1), 223–233 (2016)
17. Mellone, S., et al.: Hilbert-Huang-based tremor removal to assess postural properties from accelerometers. IEEE Trans. Biomed. Eng. **58**(6), 1752–1761 (2011)
18. Dunnewold, R.J., et al.: Ambulatory quantitative assessment of body position, bradykinesia, and hypokinesia in Parkinson's disease. J. Clin. Neurophysiol. **15**(3), 235–242 (1998)
19. Griffiths, R.I., et al.: Automated assessment of bradykinesia and dyskinesia in Parkinson's disease. J. Parkinsons Disord. **2**(1), 47–55 (2012)
20. Mera, T.O., et al.: Feasibility of home-based automated Parkinson's disease motor assessment. J. Neurosci. Meth. **203**(1), 152–156 (2012)

Why Hackers Love eHealth Applications

Rohit Goyal[1] and Nicola Dragoni[1,2]($\boxtimes$)

[1] Technical University of Denmark (DTU), Kongens Lyngby, Denmark
rgoyal.pec@gmail.com, ndra@dtu.dk
[2] Örebro University, Örebro, Sweden

Abstract. The tsunami of Internet-of-Things and mobile applications for healthcare is giving hackers an easy way to burrow deeper into our lives as never before. In this paper we argue that this security disaster is mainly due to a lack of consideration by the healthcare IT industry in security and privacy issues. By means of a representative healthcare mobile app, we analyse the main vulnerabilities that eHealth applications should deal with in order to protect user data and related privacy.

1 Introduction

In February 2015, 78.8 million of Anthem[1] customers were hacked. This has been the largest healthcare breach so far, and it opened the floodgates on a landmark year. According to the Office of Civil Rights under Health and Human Services[2], more than 113 million medical records were compromised in 2015. This security disaster was further validated by Gemalto, whose report on data breach worldwide for the first half of 2015 [6] showed that the healthcare industry is taking the lead with 84.4 million total records lost. In this paper we argue that the main reason behind this alarming situation is that security and privacy are not seriously taken into account by the healthcare IT industry yet. Security and privacy are seen only as a patch to be applied in case of discovered information leakage, never as key design features that should be considered from the very first system design phase and throughout all the healthcare IT system life cycle.

Contribution of the Paper. In order to provide a concrete example of our argument, in this paper we perform a security and privacy analysis of one of the most promising healthcare mobile system under development in Sweden, namely RAPP (Development of the Recovery Assessments by Phone Points) [7]. RAPP is a healthcare mobile and Web system for tracking the health of patients post surgery and assist them with the required care. The portal is accessible through a Web and mobile application which records patient's responses to a set of survey questions related to their recovery process. The responses are sent to the server which also provides administrative access to the healthcare organization. The RAPP architecture is very common to all the applications in the healthcare IT domain, which makes RAPP a perfect candidate for our investigation of

---

[1] https://www.anthem.com.
[2] https://ocrportal.hhs.gov/ocr/breach/breach_report.jsf.

© ICST Institute for Computer Sciences, Social Informatics and Telecommunications Engineering 2016
M.U. Ahmed et al. (Eds.): HealthyIoT 2016, LNICST 187, pp. 58–63, 2016.
DOI: 10.1007/978-3-319-51234-1_9

key security and privacy issues in healthcare mobile applications. However, it's important to stress that we are using RAPP as case study only, while the outcome of the analysis is sufficiently general to be applied to a generic healthcare mobile system, as the number of recent security and privacy breaches worldwide prove.

Methodology and Outline of the Paper. We consider a patient Bob who had surgery and has been relieved from the hospital for recovery at his home. The hospital has provided him access to the RAPP system with credentials containing his username and password. He has been asked to use the Web based interface or the application installed in his smartphone. In Sects. 2, 3, 4, 5 and 6, we look into the security implications of this system and how Bob's privacy could be compromised due to system vulnerabilities. In Sect. 7 we then sum up, providing basic security/privacy recommendations for developing healthcare IT applications.

2 Username and Password

Attack Scenario. An attacker Charlie gets the information that hospital is using 4 digit usernames and passwords for authentication. He decides to hack into the system by impersonating some users and sending rogue survey responses to the hospital administrator, thus interrupting the usual service and causing unnecessary confusion. His goal could also be a denial of service to the legitimate users who need service from the hospital. To achieve his goal, he uses a simple tool from Internet to try all combinations of 4 digit usernames and passwords.

Technical Description. In RAPP, username and password (both 4-digit numeric strings) are used for authenticating users in the system. Both have a very small search space of depth 10 and length 4 which makes them vulnerable to brute force attacks. An online tool GRC [11] estimated that 11 s would be required to break this password (with 1000 guesses per second) if the attacker knows the search space. This design choice is very weak from security standpoint.

Recommendations. It is recommended that systems use more complex passwords with greater length. The security of the passwords is greatly enhanced by use of lower and upper case characters and special symbols. A detailed guide about the password authentication can be found at OWASP Web page [1].

3 User Authentication Workflow

Attack Scenario 1. Bob decides to notify the hospital authorities about his condition after the surgery. When he tries to log in into the system, he realizes that he has forgotten his credentials. There seems to be no way for him to retrieve the forgotten password.

Attack Scenario 2. Bob's computer crashed all of a sudden due to some technical problems. He borrows his neighbor Charlie's laptop to request help from the hospital authorities. He logs in into the system and submits the survey response. He realizes that there is no option to log out from the system. He is not sure if he should return Charlie's laptop with his account logged in.

Technical Description. The systems that use password authentication need to provide a secure mechanism to the user to retrieve passwords via email or phone in case they forget it. This is important to ensure the uninterrupted service to the user. Once the user is logged in, he would want to log out from the system when he is done. The log out functionality ensures that the users can share their systems with other people which is a quite common use case.

Recommendations. The login page should provide a secure procedure for a user to retrieve or change his/her username or password, for instance by email or a security code on the mobile phone. The Web site should have logout functionality which allows users to log out from the system after each session.

4   Network Communication

Attack Scenario. Bob has a wireless Access Point configured in his house with weak or no security. An attacker Charlie who lives in the next house is always sniffing neighbors' wireless network traffic for privacy invasion. Bob opens the RAPP Website, fills the survey response and submits it. Charlie who was listening to this traffic using wireshark or similar tools would be able to see all the communication between Bob and the RAPP server. He could also replay or modify the contents of the request. In this way, the security and privacy of Bob is compromised without his awareness.

Technical Description. The RAPP client-server communication is based on API calls for logging in users and sending survey responses to the server. The following experiment has been conducted to monitor the traffic between the end points: an HTTP proxy software, known as Charles proxy [2], has been installed on the client machine listening to HTTP traffic on port 8070. The Web browser is configured to forward its HTTP traffic to localhost on port 8070. The target domain is requested by entering the URL in the address bar. The network requests to the target domain can be seen in the proxy interface along with header information and responses. It has been found that the client and server communicate over HTTP protocol. This application level protocol is inherently insecure because the communication is not encrypted. The attacker could sniff the traffic and read/modify/replay the contents of the requests and responses. The username and password are transmitted in clear text. This is a major privacy leak. Also, since the request is made on HTTP, the server is not authenticated before starting the communication. This could lead to man in the middle attack [3].

Recommendations. The communication should be protected by means of the HTTPS protocol [10], in order to have a secure channel between client and server. The major goals of the protocol are to authenticate the server and maintain privacy and integrity of the data exchanged. The server is authenticated by use of trusted Certificate Authority signed certificates providing resilience against man-in-the-middle attacks [5]. The confidentiality and integrity of the communication is achieved by encryption and use of digital signatures. The current standard for certificate keys for Public Key Infrastructure (PKI) is 2048 [12].

5   Local Storage

Attack Scenario 1. Bob is not feeling well after he got back home from surgery. He decides to notify his condition to the hospital authorities. He opens the browser and logs in into the RAPP Web portal. He fills out the survey responses but does not submit it immediately. Meanwhile, his friend Charlie visits him in his house. Charlie who is an evil neighbor opens Bob's computer and accesses his private information from the browser Local Storage. Bob's privacy gets compromised due to the saved survey responses in the browser Web storage.

Attack Scenario 2. RAPP server gets infected by malicious javascript code. When Bob loads the Website, the javascript accesses browser's local Web storage and redirects Bob to the malicious site. Bob's private data and authentication information gets compromised.

Technical Description. The local offline storage in browser (also known as Web storage) is used by Websites to save some data. This data is accessible to the user with local privileges. It has been found that the RAPP server stores the authentication ticket and the survey results in the Web storage. According to OWASP guidelines, it is recommended not to store any sensitive information in the local storage [9], as vulnerable to cross site scripting attacks [4].

Recommendations. The patient survey data can be stored in session storage rather than local storage since this information is not required for persistent use and is relevant only for the current session. As soon as the browser tab is closed, the session would be discarded. The auth token should be saved as a cookie rather than a key value pair in local storage. This because a cookie can be set with an expiry date, invalidating the user after some time. Though a cookie can be set forever until the browser cookies are cleared, it still gives more control to the administrator of the Web site. Moreover, the Web storage can be vulnerable to cross site scripting attack, thus exposing the auth token or session identifier to the attacker via malicious javascript. Also, the cookie can be set with HttpOnly flag which does not allow javascript to access it. Thus, only the target domain can access the cookie information.

6   Information Gathering

Web Server Fingerprinting. The knowledge of Web server, database, frameworks, etc..., used by a Web site gives a big advantage to the attacker to exploit known vulnerabilities in the specific version of the software or take advantage of possible misconfigurations. We did 2 simple experiments to highlight how it is easy to leak information. In the first experiment, we have pinged the RAPP URL `rapp-productiontest.nethouse.solutions`. The ping response exposes the server on which the Web application is hosted. The URL gives information about the company, location of the server and hosting service provider. In the second experiment we have configured a Charles proxy on the browser, then visited the same RAPP URL and monitored the traffic on proxy interface. The response headers for the request expose information about the Web server, Web application framework, its version, and several other similar technical details.

Recommendations. The server response headers could be disabled or obfuscated to prevent the leakage of important information. The exact steps to disable these headers would depend on the server and framework. For example, ASP.NET version header could be disabled by turning the flag "enableVersion-Header" in project's web.config to "false". By making these changes in the configuration, the developer could test the Web site again using the tools and make sure that only the necessary information is sent in the response headers.

Cookie Information. The RAPP admin portal sets the cookie when the hospital admin logs in into the portal. The authentication cookie is stored with cookie name as ".ASPXAUTH". The cookie should not reveal any information related to how it is generated. Otherwise, it makes it easier for the attacker to exploit vulnerability of a specific framework.

Recommendations. The cookie should not reveal any other information except the token. Also, MSDN documentation suggests the usage of "requireSSL" for forms posting cookie information [8]. The cookie is sent by the browser only to a secure page that is requested using an HTTPS URL.

Information Leakage. The Web site should not leak any important information related to database in the authentication step. Indeed, any specific information helps the attacker to deduce more information about the system. In one of the authentication attempts on RAPP patient Website using admin credentials, we receive the error message "Only patients can log in to the app". This message provides more information than required. An attacker can deduce that the credentials might belong to non-patient user roles. The RAPP hospital admin portal also responds with similar error messages.

Recommendations. All kinds of errors regarding log in failure should convey only the generic information e.g. "Username or password is incorrect".

7   Conclusion

The tsunami of Internet of Things and mobile applications for healthcare is not currently supported by adequate privacy and security measures, as shown by the increasing number of health data breaches in the last few years. This paper calls the healthcare IT industry to take security and privacy into serious consideration and to raise the stakes against well known security and privacy vulnerabilities. To show a concrete example of what kind of vulnerabilities an healthcare system should deal with, we have done a security and privacy analysis of the RAPP mobile healthcare system. As key outcome of this analysis, there are various basic principles and recommendations that should be taken into consideration while developing healthcare applications. We summarise these findings below.

- The user ids and passwords should follow the technical standards in terms of length, inclusion of special characters etc.
- The user log in and out should be implemented according to the use cases.
- The network communication should take place over HTTPS only.
- The authentication token should be stored safely in the browser.
- The session related information should be stored in the browser session storage.
- The Web server should not leak unnecessary information in the headers or special requests.

By considering these basic security issues from the very beginning of the application design and implementation, the final system will result significantly more secure and trustworthy, reducing the impressive numbers of successful attacks that have recently involved the healthcare industry.

References

1. OWASP: Authentication Cheat Sheet, May 2015. https://www.owasp.org/index.php/Authentication_Cheat_Sheet
2. Charles proxy, May 2015. https://www.charlesproxy.com/
3. Conti, M., Dragoni, N., Lesyk, V.: A survey of man in the middle attacks. IEEE Commun. Surv. Tutorials (2016). doi:10.1109/COMST.2016.2548426
4. Cross-site Scripting (XSS), May 2015. https://www.owasp.org/index.php/Cross-site_Scripting_(XSS)
5. Description of the Server Authentication Process During the SSL Handshake, May 2015. https://support.microsoft.com/en-us/kb/257587
6. Gemalto: First Half Review 2015, May 2015. http://www.gemalto.com/brochures-site/download-site/Documents/Gemalto_H1_2015_BLI_Report.pdf
7. Jaensson, M., et al.: The development of the recovery assessments by phone points (RAPP): a mobile phone app for postoperative recovery monitoring and assessment. JMIR mHealth uHealth 3(3), e86 (2015)
8. To, H.: Protect Forms Authentication in ASP.NET 2.0, May 2015. https://msdn.microsoft.com/en-us/library/ff648341.aspx
9. HTML5 Security Cheat Sheet, May 2015. https://www.owasp.org/index.php/HTML5_Security_Cheat_Sheet
10. HTTPS protocol, May 2015. https://en.wikipedia.org/wiki/HTTPS
11. Password strength, May 2015. https://www.grc.com/haystack.htm
12. PKI (Public Key Infrastructure), May 2015. http://searchsecurity.techtarget.com/definition/PKI

Reliable Communication in Health Monitoring Applications

Hossein Fotouhi[1(✉)], Maryam Vahabi[1], Apala Ray[1,2], and Mats Björkman[1]

[1] School of Innovation, Design, and Technology,
Mälardalen University, Västerås, Sweden
{hossein.fotouhi,maryam.vahabi,mats.bjorkman}@mdh.se
[2] ABB Corporate Research, Bangalore, India
apala.ray@in.abb.com

Abstract. Remote health monitoring is one of the emerging IoT applications that has attracted the attention of communication and health sectors in recent years. We enable software defined networking in a wireless sensor network to provide easy reconfiguration and at run-time network management. In this way, we devise a multi-objective decision making approach that is implemented at the network intelligence to find the set of optimal paths that routes physiological data over a wireless medium. In this work, the main considered parameters for reliable data communication are path traffic, path consumed energy, and path length. Using multi-objective optimization technique within a case study, we find the best routes that provide reliable data communication.

1 Introduction

The future Internet of Things (IoT) envisions a world populated by connected devices. Sensor networks are the key enablers for the future IoT applications [4]. One of the main requirements for these systems is to support coexistence of multiple applications [2]. In a health monitoring application, it is required to collect various types of measurements from patients. Each sensor or a set of sensors are supposed to measure body vital signs. For instance, ECG, heart rate and respiratory rate sensors are responsible for heart monitoring, while another set of sensors (accelerometer, gyroscope, and Magnetometer) are responsible for fall detection. Both heart and movement monitoring are very critical for elderly people. Providing a reliable communication when running concurrent health applications is of paramount importance.

In this paper, we take advantage of software defined networking (SDN) paradigm [6] in order to provide a higher level management and more flexibility for network reconfiguration. This way, we lift up network management from the infrastructure level to a higher level that can eventually improve network reliability by enabling the network agility. In SDN architecture the controller interacts with sensor nodes, and intermittently interrupts communication by updating flow tables based on the information collected from the network. We collect network and link parameters, and design a multi-objective optimization function running

© ICST Institute for Computer Sciences, Social Informatics and Telecommunications Engineering 2016
M.U. Ahmed et al. (Eds.): HealthyIoT 2016, LNICST 187, pp. 64–70, 2016.
DOI: 10.1007/978-3-319-51234-1_10

at the controller to construct new flow tables. To be concise, our contributions include: (i) designing a multi-objective SDN-based WSN, and (ii) primary evaluation of the proposed SDN-based protocol considering a use case.

The paper is organized as follows. Section 2 describes the related works on some of the existing health monitoring architectures. Section 3 mathematically formulates our system model. Section 4 evaluates the multi-objective model considering input values from a case study, and finally, Sect. 5 concludes the paper.

2 Related Works

CodeBlue [7] was designed for emergency medical care, and operates both with a small number of devices under almost static conditions, such as hospitals, as well as in ad-hoc deployments at a mass casualty site. This system architecture is very scalable with self-organising capabilities. CodeBlue supports scalability, timeliness and security, but it fails in terms of reliability.

The AID-N [3] health monitoring architecture is designed in three layers. Layer 1 consists of an ad-hoc network for collecting vital signs and running lightweight algorithms. Layer 2 includes servers that are connected to the Internet to forward information to a central server, located in Layer 3. AID-N is a real-time system architecture that fails in terms of reliability in LPWNs with unreliable links and also in networks with high sampling measurements.

The CareNet [5] builds a heterogenous network with two-tier wireless network for data sensing, collection, transmission, and processing. The intra-WBAN communication uses IEEE 802.15.4 wireless standard, while a multi-hop IEEE 802.11 wireless network provides a high performance backbone structure for packet routing. CareNet supports intra- and beyond-WBAN communications with a reasonable reliability, scalability and security. However, CareNet neglects the real-time issue in critical health monitoring applications.

The MobiHealth [8] system was designed for ambulant patient monitoring that employs cellular network, while the vital signs of the body are collected via Bluetooth and ZigBee. Thus this architecture supports both intra- and beyond-WBAN communication, however, mechanisms for security are not provided. MobiHealth provides reliability and inter-operability issues, while it fails in terms of security and data privacy.

3 System Model

In a conventional health monitoring application, the patients are equipped with a handheld device that collects the physiological data from the body sensor network. The collected data are then sent to the intended health givers (nurses and doctors) through a multi-hop network. The SDN controller will issue the rules at each forwarding nodes to route the data to the destination. We represent the communication network between the patients and the health givers by using a directed acyclic graph, $N = \{D, L\}$, where the vertices are the communication devices, $D = \{d_1, d_2, d_3, \cdots, d_{n-1}, d_n\}$, in a network, and the edges are the links between devices, $L = \{l_{d_1 d_2}, l_{d_2 d_3}, \cdots, l_{d_{n-1} d_n}\}$. Note that the links between two communication devices are labeled in order, therefore, $l_{d_i d_j}$ implies that the link is directed from device d_i to device d_j.

Sensing devices are indirectly connected to the controller which manages the network. The controller builds the flow path between the nodes in the network. A flow path (f_{d_x, d_y}) between two devices d_x and d_y is an ordered pair of links including all intermediate nodes $\{d_x, d_{x+1}, \cdots, d_{y-1}, d_y\}$, and is given by:

$$f_{d_x, d_y} = \{l_{d_x d_{x+1}}, l_{d_{x+1}, d_{x+2}}, \cdots, l_{d_{y-1} d_y}\} \tag{1}$$

It is possible to have multiple flow paths between two devices d_x, d_y. We denote each flow path as $f^k_{d_x, d_y}$, where, $k \in \{1, 2, \cdots, n\}$ and n is the number of possible paths between the two devices. In order to select the optimal flow path, we have considered three communication properties of: (*i*) *path traffic*, (*ii*) *path consumed energy* and (*iii*) *path length*. However, our proposed approach for optimal path selection can be extended with other objective functions or decision criteria.

We define the path traffic, $\rho(x, y)$, for any flow path f_{d_x, d_y} as the maximum *link traffic*, $\tau(l_{d_i d_j})$, between two neighbor nodes (d_i, d_j) in that flow path. The link traffic, $\tau(l_{d_i d_j})$, is defined by the amount of data that is exchanged between two neighbor nodes (d_i, d_j) during a predefined period of time. Assuming same packet size P_s in bit, we compute the link traffic as the number of packets P_n that is transmitted over the link during one second, and thus, $\tau(l_{d_i d_j}) = (P_n P_s)$ bps. The maximum data rate supported by the communication link provides a theoretical bound on the maximum path traffic at which packets can be transmitted through a multi-hop path. Hence, the traffic flow must be less than the supported bandwidth for any link. Assuming a flow path $f_{d_x, d_y} = \{l_{d_x, d_1}, l_{d_1, d_2}, l_{d_2, d_y}\}$, then the path traffic, $\rho(f_{d_x, d_y})$, is formulated as follows:

$$\rho(f_{d_x, d_y}) = \max(\tau(l_{d_x d_1}), \tau(l_{d_1 d_2}), \tau(l_{d_2 d_y})). \tag{2}$$

Path consumed energy, $\psi(x, y)$, for any flow path f_{d_x, d_y} is defined based on the maximum *node consumed energy*, δ, of all nodes in that flow path. The node consumed energy is the amount of energy that a node has spent. We compute the node consumed energy by $\delta(d_i) = (E_c/E_i) \times 100(\%)$, where E_i is the initial energy level at the device in mAh, and E_c is the amount of energy that is consumed. In a same way, assuming the flow path $f_{d_x, d_y} = \{l_{d_x, d_1}, l_{d_1, d_2}, l_{d_2, d_y}\}$, the path consumed energy $\psi(f_{d_x, d_y})$ of the flow path f_{d_x, d_y} is computed as:

$$\psi(f_{d_x, d_y}) = \max(\delta(d_x), \delta(d_1), \delta(d_2), \delta(d_y)) \tag{3}$$

The path length $\lambda(x, y)$ is defined as the number of *hop counts* between two devices $d_x, d_y \in D$ in the flow path f_{d_x, d_y}. The hop count is in fact the number of links in a flow path given by:

$$\lambda(f_{d_x, d_y}) = |f_{d_x, d_y}| \tag{4}$$

The performance of a health monitoring system can be assessed with regards to various communication network criteria such as end-to-end latency and link reliability. The purpose of the balancing approach presented in this work is to determine, given a network and a communication pattern, what kind of trade-off arises between chosen performance metrics when multiple paths are available between two nodes. In our SDN-based system design, the controller aims to identify a preferred path between two devices considering the three design criteria mentioned earlier, namely path traffic, path consumed energy and path length. Given a set of k paths between two devices, the problem of finding the optimal path for optimizing the three design criteria is formulated as follows:

$$\text{minimize: } [\rho(f_{d_x,d_y}), \psi(f_{d_x,d_y}), \lambda(f_{d_x,d_y})]$$
$$\text{where: } f_{d_x,d_y} = [f^1_{d_x,d_y}, f^2_{d_x,d_y}, \cdots, f^k_{d_x,d_y}] \tag{5}$$

Equation (5) is a multi-objective optimization problem. For a nontrivial multi-objective optimization problem, generally there exists no single solution that simultaneously optimizes all objectives. We define objective function set for a flow path f_{d_x,d_y} as:

$$\gamma(f_{d_x,d_y}) = \{\rho(f_{d_x,d_y}), \psi(f_{d_x,d_y}), \lambda(f_{d_x,d_y})\} \tag{6}$$

A flow path $f^*_{d_x,d_y}$ is a Pareto optimal or efficient solution iff there is no other flow path in f_{d_x,d_y}, such that:

1. $\gamma_r(f^*_{d_x,d_y}) \geq \gamma_r(f_{d_x,d_y})$ where, r = $\{1, 2, 3\}$
2. $\gamma_r(f^*_{d_x,d_y}) > \gamma_r(f_{d_x,d_y})$ at least for one $r \in \{1, 2, 3\}$

A Pareto optimal solution is obtained when none of the objective functions can be improved. After finding Pareto solutions of the multi-objective optimization problem, it is required to select the final solution as the controller needs to assign the most preferred solution. This is often a non-trivial task, and certain priorities such as application requirements should be considered.

4   Case Study

In this section, we apply our approach in a specific case study within a sample health application in a hospital, where patients' physiological data must be collected continuously. The data collection is performed by a number of physiological sensors that form a body area network. The collected data is transmitted over the wireless channel (potentially through other nodes) to a higher-tier entity (nurses or doctors) in the system. The generic system model for integrating SDN within WSNs have been explained in [1].

In this case study, we assume a scenario consisting of 16 patients and four nurses in a specific department of a hospital[1]. The patient's data should be sent

---

[1] According to the "Statista" information, there are 5,627 hospitals and 902,202 beds in the US, where it concludes that in average there are 160 beds per hospital. In a sample hospital with 10 departments, there are 16 beds per department. By applying the nurse-to-patient staffing requirement in the US (1:4), there should be four nurses per department.

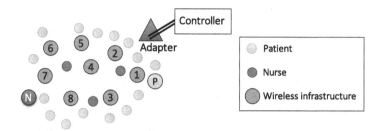

Fig. 1. Simulated network of a hospital department with 16 patients and four nurses.

Table 1. Energy consumption at each node at time t_1, $\delta_{t_1}(d_i)$.

Node number (i)	1	2	3	4	5	6	7	8
$\delta_{t_1}(d_i)$ [%]	1	5	18	10	10	15	3	7

Table 2. Traffic level at each link at time t_1, $\tau_{t_1}(l_{d_i d_j})$.

links ($l_{d_i d_j}$)	$d_1 d_2$	$d_1 d_3$	$d_2 d_4$	$d_2 d_5$	$d_3 d_4$	$d_3 d_8$	$d_4 d_5$	$d_4 d_8$	$d_5 d_6$	$d_6 d_7$	$d_7 d_8$
$\tau_{t_1}(l_{d_i d_j})$ [%]	15	15	30	30	20	25	40	50	35	40	30

through a fixed wireless infrastructure to the intended nurse. Figure 1 illustrates our network scenario, where patient "P" sends the medical information to nurse "N" in a multi-hop fashion. We explore different paths between P and N. We apply the graph transversal algorithm to the network, which results in six possible paths from P to N.

Tables 1 and 2 represent simulation parameters for the given case study at a particular time instance (t_1). We consider that the forwarding nodes employ IEEE 802.15.4 physical and MAC layers. We also assume that all forwarding nodes are similar and equipped with two AA-size batteries with a 2000 mAh capacity. The link traffic indicates the amount of data that is transmitted over the link connecting two neighbor nodes. Considering the maximum data rate 250 kbps, we compute the link traffic in percentage as $d_i - d_j = \tau(l_{d_i d_j}) \times 100/250$ – see Table 2.

Figure 2 shows all the possible paths that connects patient "P" to the nurse "N" in the scenario depicted in Fig. 1. There exist two Pareto optimal paths among the six possible paths between the patient and the nurse. The controller can choose one of the two non-dominated paths based on the application requirement. For example for delay sensitive measurements, the path with the *shortest path length* receives higher priority. However, with a larger set of Pareto optimal paths, selecting a particular path requires an additional computation in the controller. Combining multiple objectives (ρ, ψ, λ) into a single-objective scalar function would be as such computation to find a single Pareto optimal path. In some cases, it is preferable to have another path as a backup to increase network reliability.

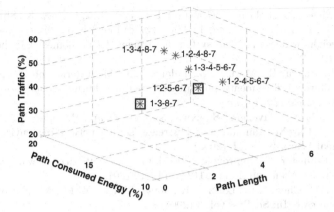

Fig. 2. Possible paths in (ρ, ψ, λ)-space, the red points indicates Pareto optimal paths. Selected routes (1-2-5-6-7 and 1-3-8-7) are among the best routes in a multi-objective function.

5   Conclusion

In this paper, we concentrated on the problem of reliable data communication in health monitoring applications using wireless sensor networks. Software defined networking paradigm provides network flexibility and on-the-fly programming in order to adjust routing path based on network and application requirements. We considered three main network parameters to select a set of optimal paths at any given time, including: (i) path traffic that considers local traffic at intermediate nodes, (ii) path consumed energy that looks at nodes' remaining battery level, and (iii) path length that counts number of hops. We considered a case study where the concept of optimal path planning is required to be done at the controller level and applied a multi-objective function to find the Pareto optimal solutions. This way, we found the most suitable paths based on network parameters at the run time and increase the reliability of data communication.

Acknowledgment. This work is funded by the Swedish Knowledge Foundation (KKS) throughout research profile Embedded Sensor System for Health (ESS-H), the distributed environments E-care@home, and Research Environment for Advancing Low Latency Internet (READY).

References

1. Fotouhi, H., Vahabi, M., Ray, A., Bjorkman, M.: SDN-TAP: an SDN-based traffic aware protocol for wireless sensor networks. In: 18th International Conference on e-Health Networking, Applications and Services (Healthcom). IEEE (2016)
2. Ganti, R.K., Ye, F., Lei, H.: Mobile crowdsensing: current state and future challenges. IEEE Commun. Mag. **49**(11), 32–39 (2011)

3. Gao, T., Massey, T., Selavo, L., Crawford, D., Chen, B.R., Lorincz, K., Shnayder, V., Hauenstein, L., Dabiri, F., Jeng, J.: The advanced health and disaster aid network: a light-weight wireless medical system for triage. IEEE Biomed. Circuits Syst. **1**, 203–216 (2007)
4. Gubbi, J., Buyya, R., Marusic, S., Palaniswami, M.: Internet of Things (IoT): a vision, architectural elements, and future directions. Future Gener. Comput. Syst. **29**(7), 1645–1660 (2013)
5. Jiang, S., Cao, Y., Iyengar, S., Kuryloski, P., Jafari, R., Xue, Y., Bajcsy, R., Wicker, S.: CareNet: an integrated wireless sensor networking environment for remote healthcare. In: ICST (2008)
6. Kim, H., Feamster, N.: Improving network management with software defined networking. IEEE Commun. Mag. **51**(2), 114–119 (2013)
7. Shnayder, V., Chen, B.R., Lorincz, K., Jones, T.R.F., Welsh, M.: Sensor networks for medical care. In: SenSys, vol. 5 (2005)
8. Wac, K., Bults, R., Van Beijnum, B., Widya, I., Jones, V., Konstantas, D., Vollenbroek-Hutten, M., Hermens, H.: Mobile patient monitoring: the MobiHealth system. In: IEEE EMBC (2009)

Security Context Framework for Distributed Healthcare IoT Platform

Orathai Sangpetch$^{(\boxtimes)}$ and Akkarit Sangpetch

Faculty of Engineering, Department of Computer Engineering,
King Mongkut's Institute of Technology Ladkrabang, Bangkok 10520, Thailand
{orathai.sa,akkarit.sa}@kmitl.ac.th

Abstract. As Internet of Things (IoT) is entering mainstream, data privacy and security in information exchange becomes a major concern and a barrier for potential adopters, especially in healthcare regime. Information from health IoT devices and services is sensitive and confidential. While many existing works have proposed enhancements and security prospects for individual devices and components in IoT ecosystems, they still do not address the underlying challenge which is the lack of sufficient security within systems. Effective security has to be built-in, not patched upon. To efficaciously tackle the challenge in distributed IoT systems, we present a security context framework which applies adaptive security contexts to properly track data of interest. The proposed solution can achieve accountability and track information propagation, involving devices, services and parties who have responsibility and potential legal liability. This could help leverage not just technical but also policy and legal aspects to enable health IoT adoption.

Keywords: Security context · Security framework · Internet of things · Cloud computing · eHealth

1 Introduction

Health and wellness is a key factor to the foundation of human capital, building strong economy. According to the UN report on the World Population Ageing [1], older population has been increasing rapidly, especially in more developed countries. There will be approximately 1,000 million older people in 2020 and double in 2050. The issue becomes one of the world's big challenges. Integrating technology, such as Internet of Things (IoT), into our lives can alleviate this challenge.

As shown in Fig. 1 for an example, a user can utilize existing wearable devices to monitor health and vital signs, such as blood pressure, heart rate, ventilation, and ECG. The monitored data will be transferred and stored at a cloud-based platform where healthcare providers or professionals can analyze and provide recommendations for users subscribing to the service. As a result, the user can spend their life independently while still receives personalized and on-demand healthcare service.

This IoT and cloud-based system mostly deals with sensitive and personal information. Cybersecurity becomes a crucial factor to effectively utilize technologies without compromising privacy. Many current IoT [8] and cloud-based solutions are not

© ICST Institute for Computer Sciences, Social Informatics and Telecommunications Engineering 2016
M.U. Ahmed et al. (Eds.): HealthyIoT 2016, LNICST 187, pp. 71–76, 2016.
DOI: 10.1007/978-3-319-51234-1_11

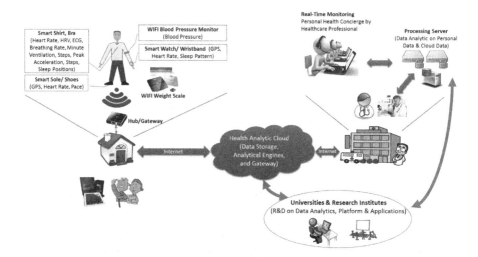

Fig. 1. An example of how to utilize internet of thing and cloud computing to provide remote and personalized healthcare service.

initially designed with security in mind. With existing threats and potential values of data, effective security cannot be just a surrounding fence like traditional security perimeter [9]; but it has to be designed within since the beginning.

In this paper, we propose a security context framework for healthcare information. The proposed framework serves as a security guideline to design the system and as a validator to evaluate security in existing systems of interest. The proposed security context should be integrated within the entire data flow since the security strength is equal to the weakest link of the flow. As illustrated in Fig. 2, if the link between the device and the gateway is compromised, the data becomes compromised even if the security in the cloud is strong. Traditional and existing data security models [4, 5] often concern with access or the implementation of individual device or software component level. This is insufficient since, if anything happens, we should be able to track the line of operations to the level of whom is responsible or at stake. Healthcare information system thus requires stronger security context than other types of system.

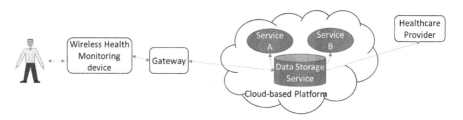

Fig. 2. A data flow example to show how personal health data gets transferred through the computing chain.

2 Security Objectives in Healthcare IoT

In order to reap the benefits of IoT technology with nominal security and privacy concern, a system that is built to manipulate healthcare information needs to satisfy at least the following security principles:

- **Authentication** is an act of verifying the truth of the credential or attributes provided.
- **Authorization** is a process to specify the access rights to resources. In this case, resources could be chunks of personal data.
- **Accountability** is an ability to trace what happens to resources of interest.
- **Confidentiality** is an act or rules to limit the access to resources of interest.
- **Integrity** is an assurance that resources of interest are accurate and trustworthy.
- **Availability** provides reliable access to resources of interest to authorized people.
- **Non-repudiation** is an implication of complete obligation to a particular contract or transaction.

3 Security Context Framework for Distributed Healthcare System

The main idea of our framework is the creation of security context associated with each resource which, in this case, is a piece of personal health information. When a piece of information is created, the associated security context should be generated automatically. The initial context is unchangeable after the creation, thereby yielding the non-repudiation property. However, at each information transfer, a device or a service can append additional context information in order to generate an audit trail, reflecting the data usage and path. We define a security context (SC) of a resource or a piece of information with an identifier X as follows.

Security Context: $SC_X = \{ACL\{action\}, Audit\{action\}\}$. The security context is essentially a pair of an access control list (ACL) and an audit list ($Audit$) of actions. An ACL specifies an action which can be acted upon the piece of information. An $Audit$ list specifies the past actions that are performed on the information associated with the context, while an action is defined as follows.

Action: action = $<actor, operation>$, where an *actor* is a pair of $<PrincipalID, StakeholderID>$. *PrincipalID* is used to identified a security principal, which can be a user, an entity, a device, or a software component. This security principal is the one who initiates the operation on the information. *StakeHolderID* represents a legal entity who is responsible for the principal, such as healthcare providers, researchers, or end users. In other words, a stakeholder is the one who owns or is responsible for the piece of information. An *operation* suggests what process is performed on the information.

In practice, when information is propagated from the source through different devices and services, not only the information but also the associated security context will be coupled together and transferred. This couple is called a *propagation context*, which is formally described as follows.

Propagation Context: $D_X = \{SC_x, information\}$ where SC_x is the security context with identifier X and this security context belongs to the enclosed information.

With our approach, information transfer or exchange among different components will be in a form of propagation context. To facilitate information propagation and exchange at scale, both *ACL* and *Audit* lists should be immutable and can only be appended when the information is processed.

For example, when a piece of information is created, the initial security context will be created. This first security context is then composed of the ÁCL and audit trail of the first action, where the actor is a pair of the information owner and the device generating the information with the *creation* operation. Concisely, *PrincipalID* will be the device ID and *StakeholderID* will be the user ID. As the information travels through the system, each principal is authenticated and checked against the security context's *ACL* to authorize whether the principal has a sufficient right to access the information. In addition, the information regarding the devices or entities processing the information during the transit should be appended to the security context's *Audit* list for traceability purpose.

4 Practicality of Deploying Security Context for IoT Applications and Discussion

In this section, we apply the security context concept proposed in Sect. 3 to verify the desirable security principles in Sect. 2. Assume that we have a healthcare system presented in Fig. 3, where user Y uses device D to monitor his health whose data will be transferred to the cloud through the gateway. Then, user Y views his data through service B. At the data creation phase, the actor will be <D, Y> and the security context's audit list will be {<<D, Y>, *Creation*>}. When the data arrives at the gateway which only transfers the data through the cloud, the security context's audit list would become {<<D, Y>, *Creation*>, <<G, Y>, *Transfer*>}. When the data reaches the cloud storage service, the security context's audit list will be {<<D, Y>, *Creation*}, <<G, Y>, *Transfer*>, <<S, C>, *Store*>}. When the user views his information through service B, the security context's audit list will be {<<D, Y>, *Creation*>, <<G, Y>, *Transfer*>, <<S, C>, *Store*>, <<B, H>, *View*>}.

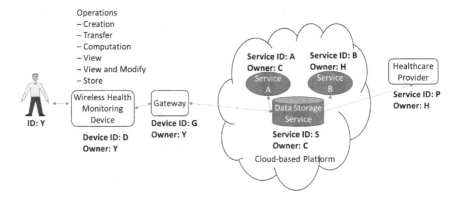

Fig. 3. An example of a security context application.

Once we construct the security context's audit list, we can consider it along with the selected technology deployed in the system in order to evaluate the security level of the given security. For example, we can use blockchain technology [7] as distributed online ledger in order to satisfy the accountability principle and the non-repudiation property as well as scalability. Currently, many financial institutions have considered to use the technology to keep track of online payment transactions.

The proposed security context can be difficult to apply to many current health monitoring devices since they are not equipped with an identification unit which can provide authorization to desired users. However, this is not an urgent concern yet. As long as the device is not sharable, we can associate a device with a user. However, it will be more secure if device providers incorporate an identification unit within the device. This can help alleviate an unauthorized use in the case of stolen devices or misusing devices to give false health data.

5 Related Works

Security and privacy issues have become a growing concern in the field of healthcare information systems and IoT. FTC report findings [2] suggest that IoT may lead to unauthorized usage of personal information by tapping into information exchange on insecure channels or through third party cloud service providers. In addition, a vulnerable device may be a potential source for staging attacks to other devices. Previous work suggests that distributed IoT approach presents unique challenges for access control due to the lack of certificate infrastructures and the need to balance the technical constraints on the range of medical devices [3]. Researchers have suggested an adaptive risk-based framework to be used to evaluate security model implementation and validate data from different IoT devices [4].

Our work has presented an extended security model for healthcare IoT. One could view IoT security framework as an extension of existing eHealth security model for exchanging EHR using cloud-based applications [5]. We propose a unified security context for medical IoT devices as well as a framework for storage and exchange of health information in the cloud. The devices also present an additional attack surface for IoT system as introduced in [6]. The security framework presented in previous works have largely focused on securing individual layers, devices, platforms, or applications independently. Our work argues that we should focus on a holistic view of security, centered on securing the pieces of information and how we should adaptively secure and track the information usage, while the information is propagating through various components and devices.

6 Conclusion

In this work, we propose an adaptive security context framework for exchanging health information in IoT ecosystem. We believe that in order to increase IoT adoption, we need to fundamentally address the challenge in data privacy and security concerning information exchange. This means we should be able to properly track and secure the pieces of information generated from healthcare IoT devices, components and services, in addition to satisfy general security principles. To achieve this, we present an information-centric approach based on usage of the proposed security context framework. The proposed framework can help ease the privacy and security concern and increase adoption in healthcare IoT system. The framework also methodically assists how to design and implement or select appropriate technologies to ensure the desired level of security in the balance of usability, device limitations, resource constraints and supporting infrastructures.

References

1. United Nations: Department of Economic and Social Affairs, Population Division: World Population Ageing 2013. United Nations Publication, New York (2013)
2. FTC Staff Report: Internet of Things: Privacy and Security in a Connected World Federal Trade Commission, Washington, DC (2015)
3. Roman, R., Zhou, J., Lopez, J.: On the features and challenges of security and privacy in distributed internet of things. Comput. Netw. **57**(10), 2266–2279 (2013)
4. Abie, H., Balasingham, I.: Risk-based adaptive security for smart IoT in eHealth. In: Proceedings of the 7th International Conference on Body Area Networks, pp. 269–275. Oslo, Norway (2012)
5. Zhang, R., Liu, L.: Security models and requirements for healthcare application clouds. In: IEEE 3rd International Conference on Cloud Computing, pp. 268–275, Miami (2010)
6. Lake, D., Milito, R., Morrow, M., Vargheese, R.: Internet of things: architectural framework for eHealth security. J. ICT Stand. **1**(3), 301–328 (2014)
7. Nakamoto, S.: Bitcoin: a peer-to-peer electronic cash system, 2009 (2012). http://www.bitcoin.org/bitcoin.pdf
8. ForeScout Technologies, Inc.: Survey Identifies Internet of Things (IoT) Security Challenges for the Connected Enterprise. Marketwired, 14 June 2016
9. Forrester: No more chewy centers: The zero trust model of information security. In: The security architecture and operations playbook for 2016

BitRun: Gamification of Health Data from Fitbit® Activity Trackers

Rachel Gawley$^{(\boxtimes)}$, Carley Morrow, Herman Chan,
and Richard Lindsay

AppAttic Ltd., Belfast, UK
{rachel, carley, herman, richard}@appattic.co.uk

Abstract. This paper presents a mobile game, BitRun that is designed to interact with Fitbit® data in the generation of the game terrain of an endless runner mobile app. By authorizing the game to interact with their Fitbit® data, a user experiences unique and personalized gameplay based on their daily activity. The aim is to use real-game mechanics to encourage users to stay engaged with their activity trackers and subsequently create positive behavior change by rewarding the user in the game for an increase their activity.

Keywords: Wearables · Gamification · Activity trackers · Fitbit® · Quantified self · Games · mHealth

1 Introduction

Within the last decade, activity tracker and wearable technologies have experienced a transformation from humble pedometers to devices that can calculate calorie burn, track sleep, record heart rate, log GPS, classify exercise types, determine elevation, etc. These devices have gone from bulky clip-on, plastic gadgets to sleek bands that are as much a fashion statement as a tracking device. The growth of activity tracker bands has increased by 67.2% from Q1 2015 to Q1 2016 [1]. The market has diversified due to the introduction of smart watches that both track activity and function as watch that connects to a mobile device. The proliferation of activity trackers has resulted in over 20% of American adults using some form of wearable technology [2].

This significant adoption of the devices provides an opportunity to harness and utilize the data to encourage healthy behaviors. Unfortunately, 32% of users stop wearing the devices within six months, and 50% after one year [3]. Our user experience suggests that the drop-off is more pronounced and is often within the first three months. This dramatically reduces the potential for the devices to be used to create initial and sustained positive behavior change or as a means of tracking surrogate markers for health. If activity trackers are to be utilized to change behavior or to track long-term health indicators, a means of keeping users engaged is required. At the same time, it would be beneficial to address the issue that activity tracker users are normally healthy and interested in their health [4] and not people who live a sedentary life and therefore could benefit the most. If trackers are used to change unhealthy behaviors, then a means to encourage and onboard users who are not already interested in the technology is

© ICST Institute for Computer Sciences, Social Informatics and Telecommunications Engineering 2016
M.U. Ahmed et al. (Eds.): HealthyIoT 2016, LNICST 187, pp. 77–82, 2016.
DOI: 10.1007/978-3-319-51234-1_12

necessary. A methodology to attract users to activity trackers, keep them engaged and encourage positive behavior change is required to be able to produce a long-term impact on health. This paper presents gamification as a means to address the afore-mentioned issues.

2 Gamification

The term 'gamification', first used in 2008, is defined as the use of game design elements in non-gaming contexts [5]. For example, point systems, competition, rewards, game mechanics, leaderboards, applying rules of play, etc. From business sales leaderboards and home chore chart through to collecting friends on Twitter, game elements have long been used in daily life to encourage productivity, behavior change and make life fun. The ubiquitous mobile app market provides the perfect opportunity to use mobile devices for gamification and thus can be attributed to its adoption as a common household term and rise in gamification within the digital space.

The aim of the project was to create an app that both encourages long-term engagement with a wearable activity tracker and also promotes healthy behavior change regarding a user's activity. In the US, 55.7% of the 2016 population is con-sidered to be a mobile gamer and this is set to reach 63.7% in 2020 [6]. Due to the popularity of mobile games and the psychological persuasive nature of video games [7] a game-first approach was taken to creating a mobile app that utilizes Fitbit®[1] [8] activity tracker data. The idea was to create a more meaningful experience for the end-user based on their activity data, potentially increasing long-term engagement, and providing a sustained platform for which positive behavior change can be achieved. Video games have in the past been noted for their impact on behavior change in a negative manner [9], however, in recent years there have been a lot of talk about their use in psychology and positive behavior change [10, 11] although there have been very little studies to test clinical effectiveness in terms of improving physical activity [12].

Well-established mobile game styles were considered as potential options to gamify wearable data. The final decision was to proceed with an "endless-runner" style game for two reasons: a runner game has parallels with the real-world idea of movement which we are encouraging and more importantly the game mechanics of this game style lends itself to being associated with activity tracker data for the purposes of gamifi-cation. The result was to produce the mobile game, BitRun that is a game-first approach to engaging users with their activity data.

---

[1] Fitbit is a registered trademark and service mark of Fitbit, Inc. BitRun is designed for use with the Fitbit platform. This product is not put out by Fitbit, and Fitbit does not service or warrant the functionality of this product.

3   BitRun: Mobile Game Using Fitbit® Data

BitRun is a mobile game available on iOS AppStore [13] and Google Play store [14] for use with Fitbit® devices to populate the game terrain a user plays. It is a runner-game, where the user plays as a ship/object on track with four lanes. A user moves left or right by tapping on the relevant sides of the mobile screen. The user must avoid the obstacles (wooden crates, boulders and road-blocks) and collect the golden rings for extra points. This gameplay is shown in Fig. 1.

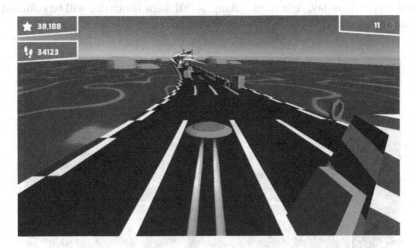

Fig. 1. BitRun gameplay

The game terrain has a pre-determined length and a user completes the game when the ship crosses the finish line. The game can be played with or without Fitbit® data. If the game is played without syncing to a Fitbit® device, the maximum possible score is 25,000 and there is the maximum number of obstacles for the user to avoid and very few rings to collect. The idea of making the game playable without interacting with Fitbit® data is to remove any barriers to onboarding a player, giving the game psychology a chance to have an effect and the competitive nature of the player to take over. When a player authorizes BitRun to interact with their Fitbit® data, a new daily terrain is generated based on the previous day's activity. The maximum achievable score will depend on the user's level of activity for the previous day. We use the previous day's worth of data, as we need a full day of data to generate the game track.

3.1   Beyond Gamification: Associating Activity Data to Terrain Generation

The game utilizes the following data in the generation of terrain: total number of active minutes and number of sedate minutes. Sedate minutes translate to obstacles: less sedate means less obstacles. The idea is to reward being active by making it easier to complete the game. Active minutes are linked to rings: the more active minutes the player has, the more rings the game will generate, with the saturation point of rings being reached at 100 active minutes. BitRun rewards activity with rings, which are then linked to additional points and thus higher score if collected. Figure 2 shows the game terrain generation screen linking active and sedate minutes to the obstacles and rings. The user also receives a bonus point for each step taken on the previous day. An additional bonus 1,000 points is also awarded to a user for simply authorizing the app to interact with their Fitbit® data. This decision was taken to encourage people to connect in the first place. Therefore, the player starts the game 1,000 points more than the number of steps they walked the previous day. As a result, taking 24,001 steps in one day will be sufficient to beat the high score of any user who has not connected their wearable device.

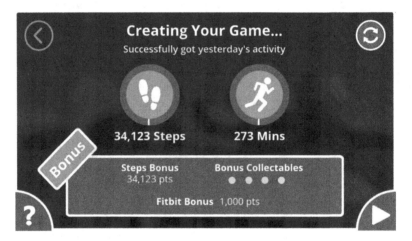

Fig. 2. Terrain, collectables and bonus point generation from Fitbit® data

3.2   Using the Traditional Leaderboard

Leaderboards feature in both video games and gamification systems. A leaderboard can activate the social, identity, challenge and feedback elements of an engaging gamification experience. Leaderboards are a key element of BitRun and there is both an in-game leaderboard, shown in Fig. 3 and a web-version of the leaderboard [15] for sharing on social media. Leaderboards create prestige and thus form a large part in motivation and engagement. The in-game leaderboard contains global all-time rankings and monthly rankings. Within a few months of release, it was evident that the leaderboard was no longer an engagement tool and became a source of demotivation for many casual users. Qualitative surveys were conducted and user dissatisfaction around the leaderboard was noted as the main reason for disengaging with the app. A small number of users with extraordinarily high number of steps had effectively set a very high entrance level to the leaderboard. This level of activity, in excess of 50,000 daily steps, is not achievable or even realistic for most users. People wanted to compete with others just like them or at least have a chance of appearing on the

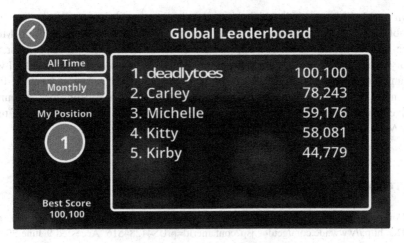

Fig. 3. BitRun in-game leaderboard

leaderboard. These are the users we need to engage, not necessarily the current leaders who are scoring in excess of 100,000 by walking over 75,000 steps in one day (approximately 37.5 miles). As a result, monthly leaderboards were introduced. This effectively resets the points every month and gives people a chance to get on the leaderboard and compete monthly. Notably, people are playing early in the month to maximize the opportunity to be number 1 even if it is for a day or two.

4   Conclusions and Future Work

With this project we created a mobile game to engage users with their activity data. The strategy was to publish the game in the Google Play and iOS app stores as a means to receive general public feedback on the concept of engagement. So far, the response has been positive and the feedback on the actual gameplay is that it looks, feels and responds like a game opposed to a gamified experience, which was our desired outcome. Our initial results indicated that leaderboards are a large portion of motivation and that a global overall leaderboard was not enough. Users become quickly disheartened trying to beat a score that was achieved by a user who walked more than 50,000 steps in a day. Therefore, we added a monthly leaderboard, which is effectively transient and resets each month. Our internal statistics indicate that people like to play the app throughout the month especially if they have had a particularly active day. Therefore, we will be introducing more granular leaderboards of weekly and daily to encourage this concept of retention with our next release.

The longer-term plan is to allow users with different types of wearables compete against each other rather than stay within the ecosystem of one type of wearable. People with a Microsoft band will be able to complete with Garmin users and people who use their phones as an activity tracker can also get involved with the game. This greatly reduces the barrier to entry for users to gamify their activity data with BitRun. Finally, BitRun was created as part of a much larger mHealth product of AppAttic's, known as MediMerge [16], which is used to collect health and wellness data from wearables, IoT, apps, and games for clinical review. We are already trialing Medi-Merge with other wearables and apps as a means of healthcare intervention for respiratory conditions. The mHealth strategy for BitRun is to run a pilot clinical trial with the game being given as an intervention for a specific cohort that would benefit from being more active. The study will focus on assessing whether BitRun does encourage positive behavior change to activity and whether this is sustained over a period of time, using MediMerge as the aggregator of the clinical data for review.

References

1. Worldwide wearables market increases 67.2% amid seasonal retrenchment, according to IDC. http://www.idc.com/getdoc.jsp?containerId=prUS41284516. Accessed 9 June 2016
2. 20 percent of Americans say they use wearable tech. http://www.nextgov.com/mobile/2015/09/20-percent-americans-say-they-use-wearable-tech/122421/. Accessed 9 June 2016
3. How the science of human behavior change offers the secret to long-term engagement. http://endeavourpartners.net/assets/Endeavour-Partners-Wearables-White-Paper-20141.pdf. Accessed 9 Sep 2016
4. Piwek, L., Ellis, D.A., Andrews, S., Joinson, A.: The rise of consumer health wearables: promises and barriers. PLoS Med. **13**(2), e1001953 (2015)
5. Deterding, S., Dixon, D., Khaled, R., Nacke, L.: From game design elements to gamefulness: defining gamification. In: Proceedings of the 15th International Academic MindTrek Conference: Envisioning Future Media Environments, 28 September 2011, pp. 9–15. ACM
6. Mobile phone gaming penetration in the United States from 2011 to 2020. http://www.statista.com/statistics/234649/percentage-of-us-population-that-play-mobile-games/. Accessed 9 Sep 2016
7. Michael, D.R., Chen, S.L.: Serious Games: Games that Educate, Train, and Inform. Muska & Lipman/Premier-Trade (2005)
8. Fitbit. http://www.fitbit.com. Accessed 9 Sep 2016
9. Bogost, I.: Persuasive Games: The Expressive Power of Videogames. MIT Press, Cambridge (2007)
10. Granic, I., Lobel, A., Engels, R.C.: The benefits of playing video games. Am. Psychol. **69**(1), 66 (2014)
11. Gibbs, M.R., Vetere, F.: Designing for social and physical interaction in exertion games. In: Nijholt, A. (ed.) Playful User Interfaces. GMSE. Springer, Heidelberg (2014). doi:10.1007/978-981-4560-96-2
12. Tabak, M., Weering, M.D., van Dijk, H., Vollenbroek-Hutten, M.: Promoting daily physical activity by means of mobile gaming: a review of the state of the art. Games Health J. **4**(6), 460–469 (2015)
13. BitRun iOS App Store. https://itunes.apple.com/gm/app/bitrun/id1050596670?mt=8l. Accessed 9 Sep 2016
14. BitRun Android. https://play.google.com/store/apps/details?id=uk.co.appattic.bitrun&hl=en. Accessed 9 Sep 2016
15. BitRun Web. http://www.bitrunapp.com. Accessed 9 Sep 2016
16. MediMerge. http://www.medimergeonline.com. Accessed 9 Sep 2016

Smartphone-Based Decision Support System for Elimination of Pathology-Free Images in Diabetic Retinopathy Screening

João Costa, Inês Sousa, and Filipe Soares[✉]

Fraunhofer AICOS, Rua Alfredo Allen 455, 4200-135 Porto, Portugal
{joao.costa,ines.sousa,filipe.soares}@fraunhofer.pt

Abstract. Diabetic Retinopathy is a Diabetes complication and the leading cause of blindness in the United States. Early detection can be accomplished by analysis of images of the retina, generally obtained by expensive fundus cameras. Recent developments allow the use of mobile ophthalmoscopes that can be adapted to smartphones to acquire these images, but the low computational power of smartphones limits the use of Computer-Aided Diagnosis systems. In this paper, an approach for automatic retinal image analysis on a smartphone is proposed, with emphasis on high sensitivity and fast computation. A set of 1200 images from the Messidor database were analyzed for extraction of features related to vessel segmentation, presence of exudates and microaneurysms. SVM and k-NN classifier models were trained with these features, resulting in a sensitivity of 87% and a specificity of 66%. An analysis of the computational performance validates the feasibility of using this approach on quad-core smartphones.

Keywords: Diabetic Retinopathy · Decision support system · Vessel segmentation · Microaneurysms · Exudates · Image processing

1 Introduction

Diabetic Retinopathy is a complication of diabetes caused by general physiological deregulation, and eventually may lead to blindness. The asymptomatic nature of the disease progression and the very large diabetic population make the implementation of extensive screening programs particularly challenging. Notwithstanding, the high effectiveness of treatment in the initial stages contributes to the great clinical value of early detection and motivate the need to improve the cost-effectiveness of screening programs.

The current gold standard for diagnosis is the acquisition of images of the retina by a retinal camera and subsequent analysis by a clinical expert. However, two challenges arise from this approach: retinal cameras are relatively expensive for wide deployment in various screening sites and are not easily transported among different screening locations; in addition, the large screening population poses a significant burden on healthcare systems, due to the necessity of manual image analysis by a scarce number of experts.

© ICST Institute for Computer Sciences, Social Informatics and Telecommunications Engineering 2016
M.U. Ahmed et al. (Eds.): HealthyIoT 2016, LNICST 187, pp. 83–88, 2016.
DOI: 10.1007/978-3-319-51234-1_13

In order to tackle the first challenge, handheld systems for acquisition of retinal images, integrating smartphone imaging capabilities with the optical principles of retinal cameras have been proposed in the literature [1,2], taking advantage of the significant image quality currently afforded by the smartphone cameras. Favourable comparisons between the image quality of these approaches to commercial retinal cameras validate their clinical potential [3].

The use of smartphone cameras as opportunistic sensors, besides significantly reducing the cost for retinal image acquisition, also allows to exploit the considerable computing power of these devices to perform automatic analysis of the acquired retinal images.

Extensive research work has been developed for the automatic detection of Diabetic Retinopathy in images acquired by traditional retinal cameras, but few address the constraints of running the proposed methods in mobile hardware. This paper describes a Decision Support System for automatic classification of retinal images according to the presence of Diabetic Retinopathy, with emphasis on fast computation and high sensitivity in detecting pathological cases, for use in mobile devices.

2   Methods

A total of 1200 images from the publicly available Messidor database [4] are used. The images were acquired by a Topcon TRC NW6 retinograph with a 45° field of view and saved in 8-bit color depth uncompressed TIFF format, with a resolution of 2240×1488 pixels, 1440×960 pixels and 2304×1536 pixels.

The ground truth for this database considers four different Retinopathy grades: R0 (no Retinopathy signs) and R1, R2 and R3, in ascending order of severity. Since our goal is to exclude images without signs of Diabetic Retinopathy, all images with grade above R0 were considered as presenting this pathology - from the 1200 images, 654 present Diabetic Retinopathy and 546 do not.

Classification uses three specific retinal structures detected by image analysis methods: retinal vessels, microaneurysms and exudates. The proposed methods are implemented in C++, using the OpenCV library.

From the original input image, the green channel of the RGB color space is often used for the main processing steps. The reason for this decision is the superior contrast of this channel, in opposition to the significant oversaturation of the red channel and undersaturation of the blue channel.

2.1   Vessel Segmentation

A significant increase in the area of vessels is indicative of late stage Diabetic Retinopathy, where neo-vascularization often occurs.

The first step of this method removes the background variations of the retina, by subtracting the original green channel image by its median filtered version. Grayscale morphological operations are then used to evidentiate the vessels: a top hat transform will subtract the image with a morphological opened version of itself. The result is thresholded and small connected components are removed in order to obtain the final vessel segmentation.

2.2 Microaneurysm Lesions

Microaneurysms appear as small red dots in the retinal images and are the earliest sign of Diabetic Retinopathy. Microaneurysms present specific characteristics in retinal images that are suitable for detection: small size, circular shape and hypointensity in relation to the background. These features can be leveraged by image processing methods to evidentiate these structures.

An approach similar to the one proposed by Zhang et al. [5] was employed to extract microaneurysm regions from the image. An inverted 2D Gaussian kernel is used to perform template matching in the original green channel image. This kernel emulates the distribution of intensities of a microaneurysm in a retinal image and is modeled by the Eq. (1).

$$F(x,y) = -e^{-\left(\frac{x^2}{2\sigma_x^2} + \frac{y^2}{2\sigma_y^2}\right)} \tag{1}$$

In order to account for different microaneurysm sizes, different σ values are used for the kernel. The result of the template matching is thresholded and each connected component will constitute a detected microaneurysm. Since the vessels are the regions of frequent false positives, the vessel mask is used to exclude those erroneous detections (see Fig. 1).

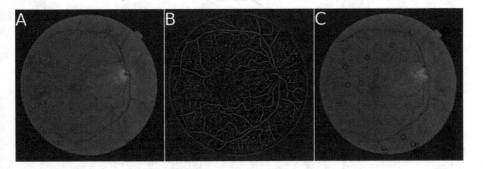

Fig. 1. Steps of the microaneurysm extractor: (A) Green channel image; (B) Result of correlation with inverted Gaussian kernel; (C) Candidates obtained by thresholding the correlation image (marked with black circles).

2.3 Segmentation of Exudate Lesions

Exudates are yellow structures that often appear in the retina as a result of the progression of Diabetic Retinopathy. Detection of these lesions is performed using morphological operations. The green channel of the retinal image is initially equalized using adaptive histogram equalization and a morphological closing operation is then applied. A local standard deviation filter is used in the resulting image - this filter will compute, for each pixel, the standard deviation of the pixel neighbourhood. The output of the filter is thresholded, and will constitute the exudates segmentation.

2.4   Classification

The area of detected vessels, the number of detected microaneurysms and the area of exudates are used as features for the decision support system. Both area values are normalized in respect to image resolution. Support Vector Machines (SVM) and k-Nearest Neighbors (k-NN) classifiers are used to classification models based on the aforementioned features. The SVM classifier uses a Radial Basis Function (RBF) kernel, with $\gamma = 1.0$ and $C = 0$. The k-NN classifier uses $k = 11$.

3   Results

The performance of the trained classifier models was evaluated using 10-fold cross validation, with sensitivity and specificity used as performance metrics. For the SVM model a sensitivity of 87% and a specificity of 66% is achieved and for the k-NN model the sensitivity is 83% and the specificity is 64%. The ROC curve for both classifiers is represented in Fig. 2. An AUC of 0.85 was registered for the SVM model and a AUC of 0.82 for the k-NN model.

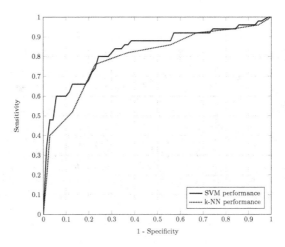

Fig. 2. Comparison of the ROC curves using SVM and k-NN classifiers.

To assess the feasibility of running the proposed methods on low power devices, the execution time of each stage was measured. The results are summarized in Table 1. All results were obtained for a smartphone with a Quad Core 2.5 GHz Snapdragon 801 CPU. The running time for the model based prediction is very low and for that reason was not considered.

Table 1. Average running time of the image processing methods.

Method	Running time (s)
Vessel segmentation	0.32 ± 0.07
Microaneurysm detection	3.02 ± 0.29
Exudates detection	3.46 ± 0.28

4 Discussion

Some studies [6,7] in the literature propose the automatic analysis of images from the Messidor database considering the four class ground truth for their results and therefore are not directly comparable. However, the work of Sánchez et al. [8] and Antal et al. [9] also uses this database with a two class prediction, considering a Diabetic Retinopathy present/absent classification.

Comparable results are obtained in these studies, in particular a sensitivity of 92% and a specificity of 50% are reported in [8], while in [10], a sensitivity of 96% and a specificity of 51% are disclosed.

Prasanna et al. [10] reports an average sensitivity of 86% and an AUC of 0.84 for pathology detection in images from the Messidor database, but these results are relative to only a portion of the database (400 out of the 1200 images) and it is not clear how the two classes were obtained from the original four class ground truth.

Execution time has been reported in [8], and for the several stages it is estimated to be under 3 min, for a desktop computer. In [11], the execution time is 31 s for an unrooted Galaxy S GT-I9000 device. Our results compare favorably with these, with a total average running time of under 7 s achieved on a smartphone. Experimentally, on a computer we found execution time to be 5 to 8 times inferior.

5 Conclusion

An approach for automatic exclusion of pathology-free cases by analyzing the retinal images, suitable for running in low-powered devices, is described in this paper. The execution time of the proposed methods is very low, which fits the use case of mobile applications. The classification results attest its competitiveness against other solutions with AUC of 0.85, specially considering the low number of features used.

In future work, we intend to validate the proposed method in images acquired using the smartphone and an optical adapter.

Acknowledgements. We would like to acknowledge the financial support obtained from North Portugal Regional Operational Programme (NORTE 2020), Portugal 2020 and the European Regional Development Fund (ERDF) from European Union through the project Symbiotic technology for societal efficiency gains: Deus ex Machina (DEM), NORTE-01-0145-FEDER-000026.

The experimental data were kindly provided by the Messidor program partners (see http://www.adcis.net/en/DownloadThirdParty/Messidor.html).

References

1. Haddock, L.J., Kim, D.Y., Mukai, S.: Simple, inexpensive technique for high-quality smartphone fundus photography in human and animal eyes. J. Ophthalmol. **2013** (2013). Article ID 518479
2. Myung, D., Jais, A., He, L., Blumenkranz, M.S., Chang, R.T.: 3D printed smartphone indirect lens adapter for rapid, high quality retinal imaging. J. Mob. Technol. Med. **3**(1), 9–15 (2014)
3. Russo, A., Morescalchi, F., Costagliola, C., Delcassi, L., Semeraro, F.: Comparison of smartphone ophthalmoscopy with slit-lamp biomicroscopy for grading diabetic retinopathy. Am. J. Ophthalmol. **159**(2), 360–364 (2015)
4. Decenciere, E., Zhang, X., Cazuguel, G., Laÿ, B., Cochener, B., Trone, C., Gain, P., Ordónez-Varela, J.R., Massin, P., Erginay, A., et al.: Feedback on a publicly distributed image database: the messidor database. Image Anal. Stereology **33**, 231–234 (2014)
5. Zhang, B., Wu, X., You, J., Li, Q., Karray, F.: Detection of microaneurysms using multi-scale correlation coefficients. Pattern Recogn. **43**(6), 2237–2248 (2010)
6. Venkatesan, R., Chandakkar, P., Li, B., Li, H.K.: Classification of diabetic retinopathy images using multi-class multiple-instance learning based on color correlogram features. In: 2012 Annual International Conference of the IEEE on Engineering in Medicine and Biology Society (EMBC), pp. 1462–1465. IEEE (2012)
7. Chandakkar, P.S., Venkatesan, R., Li, B.: Retrieving clinically relevant diabetic retinopathy images using a multi-class multiple-instance framework. In: SPIE Medical Imaging. International Society for Optics and Photonics (2013)
8. Sánchez, C.I., Niemeijer, M., Dumitrescu, A.V., Suttorp-Schulten, M.S., Abramoff, M.D., van Ginneken, B.: Evaluation of a computer-aided diagnosis system for diabetic retinopathy screening on public data. Invest. Ophthalmol. Vis. Sci. **52**(7), 4866–4871 (2011)
9. Antal, B., Hajdu, A.: An ensemble-based system for microaneurysm detection and diabetic retinopathy grading. IEEE Trans. Biomed. Eng. **59**(6), 1720–1726 (2012)
10. Prasanna, P., Jain, S., Bhagat, N., Madabhushi, A.: Decision support system for detection of diabetic retinopathy using smartphones. In: 2013 7th International Conference on Pervasive Computing Technologies for Healthcare (PervasiveHealth), pp. 176–179. IEEE (2013)
11. Bourouis, A., Feham, M., Hossain, M.A., Zhang, L.: An intelligent mobile based decision support system for retinal disease diagnosis. Decis. Support Syst. **59**, 341–350 (2014)

Improving Awareness in Ambient-Assisted Living Systems: Consolidated Data Stream Processing

Koray İnçki[1]([⊠]) and Mehmet S. Aktaş[2]

[1] Computer Engineering Department,
Adana Science and Technology University, Adana, Turkey
kincki@adanabtu.edu.tr
[2] Computer Engineering Department,
Yıldız Technical University, Istanbul, Turkey
aktas@yildiz.edu.tr

Abstract. Ambient Assisted Living (AAL) aims providing a quality of life to elderly for sustaining their lives without constant supervision. The technology developments enabled devices with more processing power, longer battery life and more advanced sensor capabilities. Internet of Things (IoT) is a phenomenon that allows seamless interconnection of very small devices over Internet; bringing new opportunities for AAL solutions. AAL systems equipped with IoT devices will generate vast amount of data in short time, thus a big data problem to mangle. This study proposes a simulation infrastructure that allows researchers to create their own AAL scenarios without real devices, and a system architecture to tackle the big data problem that is inferred by utilization of IoT in AAL systems. In order to understand feasibility of the architecture we conduct a performance experiment, in which we increase the number of messages that the system can handle per second. The resulst of the experiment are promising.

Keywords: Ambient-Assisted Living · Internet of Things · Big data · Kafka · Complex-event processing · Stream processing

1 Introduction

Internet of Things (IoT) is a new term that implies utilization of a collection of enabling technologies in a seamless and coherent way for interconnection of "things" in our lives. When K. Ashton conied the term in 1999 [1], he suggested to interconnect sensors and actuator devices so that they don't require the intervention of human beings in order to cooperate. The devices that are equipped with IoT capabilities can execute the sensing and acting duties they are predestined to, whilst they cooperate with devices from far away locations through Internet connection capability. These devices are usually resource constraint devices which lack enough processing power, and storage space for running resource-hungry applications, such as processing high volumes of data.

One can notice the time delay between the mass proliferation of the phenomenon and the first time it was introduced in to the literature. We believe that the reason behind this delay was the lack of standardization and open-source community support.

© ICST Institute for Computer Sciences, Social Informatics and Telecommunications Engineering 2016
M.U. Ahmed et al. (Eds.): HealthyIoT 2016, LNICST 187, pp. 89–94, 2016.
DOI: 10.1007/978-3-319-51234-1_14

The implementation momentum of the technology has been increasing since the adoption of standardization efforts in certain technology areas, such as communication and networking. Constrained Application Protocol (CoAP) [2] is a soon-to-be standard application layer protocol for Constrained Resource Environments (CoRE) [3]. The resource constraint devices, which are installed with resource-efficient operating systems such Contiki-OS, have more support for CoAP-like network protocols.

AAL is devised to improve quality of life for elderly people [5]. Its main purpose is to enable elderly people to live in their own houses according to their own life styles while still maintaining their well-being and safety. The utilization of IoT technologies is an ongoing discussion in the AAL community, because it opens up new opportunities for various and diverse application scenarios [4]. AAL systems generally rely on powerful backend systems for analyzing data and decision making; and the decisions that such systems make are as reliable and usable as the real-timeliness of the decisions. Increasing number of IoT systems in AAL systems will generate mass streams of data to process in a very short amount of time. Therefore, we need to employ data stream processing approaches to effectively asses such big data on run time. Real-time data stream processing has to meet certain criteria in order to retain the real-time properties of the data. We propose to integrate the complex-event processing technology with real-time big data stream processing technology such that an architectural framework will incorporate best features of both technologies to tackle real-time big data processing problem in AAL-IoT systems.

2 Background

IoT. IoT describes coherent collaboration of a set of enabling technologies. Those enabling technologies are ubiquitous communication through IP-based networking, ambient intelligence through sensor and actuator capabilities, unique identification through URI based naming services [2]. These concepts impact the proliferation of this technology tremendously. Ubiquitous communication allows for accessing the things anytime from anywhere, thus enabling a seamless interoperation between 'things'. Ambient intelligence capabilities provide the 'things' to capture physical phenomenon going on around them through sensor features, and enables them to process the data gathered from their environment. Unique identification feature not only help to authenticate the devices but also promotes heterogeneity in the manufacturing parties of those devices.

AAL. Common features of AAL applications are providing health support, safety, independence, mobility and social interaction. These devices are frequently utilized in closed loop service model, in which data produced by devices are gathered for deducing intelligent conclusions for the well-being of the elderly person (e.g., reminding to take a pill, to alert closest emergency personnel in case of abrupt changes in the person's vital signs). With the introduction of IoT technologies, those devices are becoming more reliant on service-oriented interfaces, which enable care-givers remotely monitor the person.

CoAP. CoAP is designed to provide HTTP-like communication paradigm for resource-constraint devices [2]. It enables communication between endpoints by using a request/response messaging model. It mainly designed according to RESTful guidelines, so it supports methods like GET, PUT, POST, and DELETE. Its low overhead and simplicity make it suitable for constraint resource environments. Endpoints behave either as client or a server in a request/response message model. Erbium [6] is a C implementation of the standard for Contiki-OS [7], and Californium [8] is a Java implementation for host systems.

CEP (Complex-Event Processing). An event can be described as an occurrence or action that changes the state, so that we need to take reaction. Complex-events can be described as a collection of simple events. Simple events constitute complex events according to various relations, such as timing, location, context, etc. Complex-event processing helps designers of information systems to make more intelligent decisions based on simple events occurring in a system. Esper [10] is an open-source implementation CEP engine, which has a particular programming language to describe simple events and patterns of relations amongst those so as to generate complex-events.

Stream Processing. Results of processing real-time data might affect operation of various applications, and such critical information must not be altered, neither can it be neglected. For example, an alarm generated by a heart-rate monitoring system must be immediately intercepted and care-givers must be notified at real-time. Kafka [9] is a log-based stream processing tool that allows processing real-time data in-memory caches, which allows for very fast processing. It also supports exactly-once processing paradigm, which guarantees processing a data once and only once in the system. Such reliable data processing is crucial for AAL systems in order to provide a reliable service to the elderly people.

3   Improving Awareness Through Stream Processing

Closed-loop service for AAL systems might be sufficient for ultimate well-being of elderly people. In such a system, the system might remind the patient to take some pill. On the other hand, if AAL systems are improved with decision making mechanisms, then human effort and error for acting on certain abnormal conditions would be improved. In certain situations, simple data coming from individual sensor devices can be aggregated to make more informed decisions. For example, increased blood pressure rate and falling data of an elderly might mean that the person is having a heart-attack. Here, we propose our solution architecture for such health related decision scenarios.

Figure 1 shows three sensors; blood-pressure rate, fall sensor, and body temperature sensor; which are implemented as applications that run on Contiki-OS [7]. Each sensor application is loaded onto a mote (a wireless node), and motes are simulated on Cooja simulation environment [7]. Motes are preinstalled with Erbium CoAP library, by which each mote acts as a CoAP server for serving its sensor data. CoAP client is implemented in Java by utilizing Californium open-source library [8]. Border router enables CoAP clients access to servers through IPv6 based unique addresses. CoAP protocol facilitates accessing sensor values as services provided in accordance with

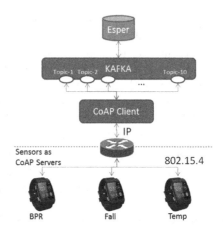

Fig. 1. Architecture for real-time stream processing of health data.

RESTful APIs. This feature of the framework allows us to insert any type of sensor device produced by any manufacturer, provided that the device implements CoAP server capabilities as before.

CoAP continuously updates clients with new sensor data at server devices by OBSERVE method, which allows us to establish a reliable monitoring architecture for AAL systems. Servers send data to clients in a quadruplet that is composed of *{SensorId, Value, Timestamp, SensorType}*. Each sensor might have a particular value range and period of sending update messages might change as well.

CoAP Client receives the sensor data from servers and relays them to appropriate *Topic* in Kafka In-Memory processing system. Having a logging mechanism such as Kafka improves the reliability of our approach, because Kafka guarantees the processing of each data once and only once during its lifetime. Moreover, it performs its operations in cache so that it improves the temporal performance of the overall system. As it can be seen from Fig. 1, CoAP client publishes updates to particular topics in Kafka, and then Esper engine receives those updates through the subscription mechanism provided by Kafka. The data published by CoAP client constitute simple events for the Esper engine.

4   Experiment and Evaluation

In order to understand the performance of proposed solution, we have to conduct an experiment on a sample IOT system. To achieve this, we increased the number of message load on the system to assess the system performance.

Complex-events generated by Esper engine represent the emergency actions to be taken on abnormal situations in well-being of a person. The scenarios we have implemented are fictional: **Heart Attack Scenario:** When the arteries to the heart get blocked or rupture, this starts affecting the hearth's functioning. This prevents the normal circulation of the blood in the body. We identify the symptoms of heart attack as follows:

(a) Sudden increase in body temperature, (b) Sudden increase in blood rate, (c) Sudden loss of balance or coordination. **Stroke Scenario:** One can think of a stroke like the brain's version of a heart attack. When arteries to the brain become blocked or rupture, they start killing brain cells and sometimes causing permanent brain damage and even paralysis. We identify the symptoms of stoke as follows: (a) Sudden loss of balance or coordination, (b) Sudden shortness of breath and increase in heart rate. Those scenarios can be expressed in Esper engine by using EPL format in Table 1 follows.

Table 1. Formal representation of rules in complex event processing for abnormal health situations

Rule ID	Formal Representation	Description
Rule 1	**ON PATTERN** ((((Body_Temperature $(\tau \rceil > \zeta$ TEMPRATURE) $\wedge$ (Blood_rate $(\tau \rceil > \zeta$ BLOOD_RATE) $\wedge$ (HAS_FALLEN node $(\tau \rceil > \zeta$ 0)) **DO ACTION (invoke** heart_attack_procedure)	If disjunction of Body_Temperature, Blood_Rate, and the Fallen Status level exceeds threshold value within a specified time period τ, then we consider this situation as Heart Attack Situation
Rule 2	**ON PATTERN** ((Blood_Rate $(\tau \rceil > \zeta$ BLOOD_RATE) $\wedge$ (Noise_Level node $(\tau \rceil > \zeta$ NOISE_LEVEL) $\wedge$ (HAS_FALLEN node $(\tau \rceil > \zeta$ 0)) **DO ACTION (invoke** stroke_procedure)	If disjunction of Blood_Rate, Noise_Level and the Fallen Status level exceeds threshold value within a specified time period τ, then we consider this situation as Stroke Attack Situation

As it can been seen in Table 1, if the certain collection of simple events collected from IoT devices are above predefined threshold values, then the system detects the Complex Events and invokes the relevant procedures.

We performed Load Testing by increasing the message load within a time period to measure system performance. We increased the number of events per second starting from 50 msgs to 700 msgs. We measured the latency of the messages in each component of the system. Up to 600 messages/second, the components of the system showed negligible latency (in the order of seconds). However, the results show that after 600 message load, the latency for the publish-subscribe message bus (Kafka) has increased to a peak value that was over 400 ms. It was clear that additional Kafka node should be included into the system to avoid the bottlenecks in message overload. Based on performance evaluation results, processing overhead of the introduce system was acceptable for our current system.

These results indicate that the performance overhead is negligible until after 600 msgs/sec on the system. If there is need for message load of 600 msgs/sec we recommend that there needs to be another Kafka (Publish/Subscribe) node in the system.

5 Conclusion

Real-time processing of sensitive data as health data requires special solutions, as such a process necessitates a fast and reliable information system to process the data. In this paper, we proposed an architecture that integrates open-source software for complex-event processing and stream processing, which promises to seamlessly analyze real-time data flowing from health sensors from an elderly person. Our experiment on open-source simulation environment demonstrates the validity of our approach based on collected data. We believe using such open-source, community supported software for AAL purposes will promote development of new solution architectures.

References

1. Ashton, K.: That 'Internet of Things' thing. RFID J. **22**(7), 97–114 (2009). http://www.rfidjournal.com/articles/view?4986
2. IEEE Constrained Application Protocol Standard. https://tools.ietf.org/html/rfc7252
3. IETF Constrained RESTful Environments Charter. https://datatracker.ietf.org/wg/core/charter/
4. Gubbi, J., Buyya, R., Marusic, S., Palaniswani, M.: Internet of Things (IoT): a vision, architectural elements, and future directions. Elsevier Future Gener. Comput. Syst. J. **29**(7), 1645–1660 (2013)
5. Costa, R., Carneiro, D., Novais, P., et al.: Ambient assisted living. In: Springer 3rd Symposium of Ubiquitous Computing and Ambient Intelligence, Salamanca, Spain (2008)
6. Kovatsch, M., Duquennoy, S., Dunkels, A.: A low-power CoAP for Contiki. In: Proceedings of the 8th IEEE International Conference on Mobile Ad-hoc and Sensor Systems. IEEE, Valencia (2011)
7. Dunkels, A.: Contiki - a lightweight and flexible operating system for tiny networked sensors. In: 29th Annual IEEE International Conference on Local Computer Networks, Florida, USA (2004)
8. Kovatsch, M., Lanter, M., Shelby, Z.: Californium: scalable cloud services for the internet of things with CoAP. In: 4th International Conference on Internet of Things, MA, USA (2014)
9. Kreps, J., Narkhede, N., Rao, J.: Kafka: a distributed messaging system for log processing. In: ACM NetDB 2011, Athens, Greece (2011)
10. Esper Open-Source Complex-Event Processing Engine. http://www.espertech.com/esper/

Beyond 'Happy Apps': Using the Internet of Things to Support Emotional Health

Jeanette Eriksson$^{(\boxtimes)}$ and Nancy L. Russo

Computer Science Department, IoTaP Research Center, Malmö University,
Nordenskiöldsgatan 1, Malmö, Sweden
{jeanette.eriksson,nancy.russo}@mah.se

Abstract. Emotions and physical health are strongly related. A first step towards emotional well-being is to monitor, understand and reflect upon one's feelings and emotions. A number of personal emotion-tracking applications are available today. In this paper we describe an examination of these applications which indicates that many of the applications do not provide sufficient support for monitoring a full spectrum of emotional data or for analyzing or using the data that is provided. To design applications that better support emotional well-being, the full capabilities of the Internet of Things should be utilized. The paper concludes with a description of how Internet of Things technologies can enable the development of systems that can more accurately capture emotional data and support personal learning in the area of emotional health.

Keywords: Internet of Things · Emotion · Emotion-tracking applications

1 Introduction

Very little research has been conducted on the extension of Internet of Things (IOT) systems to include emotion detection. Similar to how wearable health tracking devices connected to the IOT can track physical metrics such as steps and heart rate for personal use or in a healthcare context, data relating to emotions can also be tracked using wearable devices, mobile applications, and other sensors as part of the IOT.

Emotions influence health both directly (through physiological responses) and indirectly through changes in decisions and behavior [1, 2]. Although the majority of studies on emotions and health have been focused on cardiovascular disease, indicating that individuals who can better regulate emotions are at a significantly lowered risk for heart disease [3], there is growing recognition of a more general relationship between emotions and health [4].

Emotions are complex states, which have neurological, physiological, cognitive, and behavioral aspects [5]. Emotion-detecting applications have been developed to sense emotion through voice patterns, facial expressions, physiological sensors (ECG), and brain wave sensors (EEG). While acknowledging the complex nature of emotion, some researchers believe that the best way to determine what an individual experiencing an emotion actually feels is to use self-reporting [6]. That approach is what we see in the personal emotion tracking applications available today.

© ICST Institute for Computer Sciences, Social Informatics and Telecommunications Engineering 2016
M.U. Ahmed et al. (Eds.): HealthyIoT 2016, LNICST 187, pp. 95–100, 2016.
DOI: 10.1007/978-3-319-51234-1_15

To understand how personal tracking of emotions is currently enabled and how the results are used, we examined consumer-focused, personal emotion-tracking applications. To structure the evaluation, a framework developed to compare personal informatics applications was used [7]. Following this assessment of the current state of emotion-tracking applications, we discuss additional considerations that should be addressed in the design of IOT systems that address emotional well- being. The paper concludes with a discussion of implications for the design and development of emotion-sensing IOT systems and identification of areas that are particularly in need of additional research.

2   Analysis of Self-reporting Emotion Apps

To explore existing consumer applications that support self-reporting of emotions, keywords "happiness", "emotions", "mood", "mood tracker", and "feelings" were used to search for apps on Google Play and the App Store. In addition, we searched forums on the internet where various types of emotion apps were discussed. The selection criteria was for the application to have as it primary function the ability to track and individually reflect on emotions. (This excluded, for example, applications used to track mood as a way of predicting menstrual cycles.)

The search resulted in 92 apps of which 34 were disregarded because they did not work, required the login associated with a therapy group, turned out not to have emotion tracking as a primary task or were no longer available. (A complete list of the applications can be obtained from the authors.) Only one app worked with a separate hardware sensor (galvanic skin response) but the sensor is no longer available for purchase so the app was therefore not included in the analysis. It is interesting to note that very few (only about 30%) of the developers of the applications in this study claim to be grounded in psychological research or practice.

The remaining 57 apps were installed and analysed according to Ohlin et al.'s [7] classification system which includes a total of 9 dimensions on which to evaluate the applications: (1) selection of data to collect, (2) temporality of collection, (3) support during manual entry, (4) data collection control, (5) form of goal setting, (6) data analysis control, (7) form of comparison, (8) subject(s) of comparison and (9) appraisal. The dimensions can be viewed from the perspective of the type of support provided, and this more parsimonious structure will be used to frame our evaluation of emotion-tracking applications. Collection support deals with how to support the user to collect data (dimensions 1–4), while procedural support is about how the app supports users in their daily use of the app such as by providing notifications to collect data and by providing encouragement (dimensions 4–7). The third type of support, analysis support, is about how the users can be supported when analysing and reflecting on the data (dimension 6–9).

2.1 Collection Support

Collection support refers to how data is collected and how the collection is made easier for the users. In most of the apps there are predefined emotions to choose from in form of symbols and/or words. In some of the apps it is possible to make a selection of a subset of emotions to use for reporting. Half of the apps also allow for user defined data through adding free text to describe a feeling. A few apps allow for more customization, for example T2 Mood tracker and InFlow.

As mentioned only one of the apps originally identified, EMet – emotional meter, has support for hardware sensors that could collect emotions continuously. However this sensor is no longer available so the application was not included in the analysis. All the other apps collect emotion data as single entries by the users. Only one quarter of the apps analysed allow the user to edit a previous entry.

To represent emotions most of the apps use emoji of different kinds. A couple of the apps use an affect grid [8] where you position your emotion in one of four quadrants depending on whether you feel a pleasant or unpleasant feeling in combination with high or low arousal.

As the apps rely on solely self-reporting, the users need to be reminded to record an emotion. Surprisingly, less than half of the apps contains some kind of notification. How the user is notified or prompted varies. Most of the reminders are simple notifications in the mobile phone's notification field. Some apps use widgets that are activated and prompt the users to record their emotions when opening the phone. It is in many cases possible to tailor when the notification should show up. Only four apps use random notifications.

What we can learn from the analysis of the apps in terms of data collection support is that it is important to represent emotions in a way the individual user finds appropriate. The representation must be nuanced and reflect the user's emotion. A customizable combination of words and symbols might be a good way to move forward. Another aspect to consider is how the representation of the emotions may evolve in line with the user's understanding of their own emotions.

2.2 Procedural Support

Procedural support assists in the daily use of the application, aiding in integrating the application with the user's lifestyle and achieving desired outcomes. In their evaluation of general apps for personal informatics (PI), Ohlin et al. [7] identified procedural support as generally underdeveloped. The same can be said for emotion- tracking apps. There are only a few attempts to combine activities with emotion tracking. For example Activity Mood Tracker makes the user track her emotion before and after a pleasant activity to make the user reflect on the potential change.

Goal setting is considered important in PI, but in the emotion apps goals are sparsely considered. Moodlytics makes an attempt by letting the user choose a goal for how long she wants to be happy every day. This kind of goal is very crude in the context of emotions where it could potentially lead to a more negative state if the goal is not achieved.

When it comes to data analysis control none of the apps try to prompt the user to look back at the reported values. It is completely up to the user if and when to reflect on the reported emotions.

It is common in PI to compare the results with self and others. In emotion apps it is mainly oneself that is the subject of comparison. An exception is Emotion Sense. In Emotion Sense the user has to answer a set of questions that are evaluated and compared to statistics about the general population.

Rather than setting goals as quantifiable measures, there may be better ways to direct emotion-related activities such as through describing an overall ambition or desired state. The notifications that exist in the reviewed apps are rather blunt. A more context-aware approach to providing notifications should be considered. In addition the users should be prompted to reflect on the day to be able to learn what made them feel like they did.

2.3   Analysis Support

Analysis support is neglected in most of the apps. The apps display the data in different ways and in different historical time spans or in calendars, but there is not any support to interpret the data and guide the user as to what the data may mean. As mentioned above, Emotion Sense interprets a set of questions and presents it as insight of who you are, but there is no transparency of how this is done which both leads to a lack of trust and prevents learning from it.

Sharing data with friends or therapists is quite common in these emotion-tracking applications. This can be done in different ways and with different mediums such as e-mail, Twitter, Facebook etc. Most of the interaction and appraisal take place outside of the app. MoodPanda has taken another direction and has an internal forum where users can respond to other users' emotions and give them a virtual hug.

The take away regarding analysis support is that there is a need to visualize a bigger picture where the user's emotions are put in context, possibly by comparing with other users in a clever, non-critical way. There is also a need to help the user interpret the data. The ability to share the data, if desired, to receive social support is another important aspect of these applications.

3   Additional Considerations for Emotion-Sensing Apps

The same types of metrics, tracking, and support structures cannot be taken directly from personal informatics applications and applied without modification to emotion tracking applications. There are several significant differences between 'emotion management' and typical personal informatics (also called quantified self) applications. Three of these – levels of abstraction, ethical issues, and goal setting – are discussed below.

3.1 Levels of Abstraction in Measuring Emotion

When evaluating emotion, we are not attempting to capture just one measurable physiological state such as heart rate or one value captured by sensors on a device. Emotion involves a range of responses from the neurobiological to the behavioral. The context and other factors specific to the individual may influence the subjective feeling of the emotion experienced. Thus an individual's emotional state at any particular moment reflects and is influenced by a broad range of factors. To truly capture an emotional state, it may be necessary to combine neurological, physiological, and contextual data on an on-going basis. Environmental factors such as traffic, temperature and noise level may contribute to an individual's emotional state. Location of the user, the proximity of others, and life events and activities may influence emotion. A simple periodic self-reporting of emotional state may be useful in tracking how the user feels over time, but does not address the deeper issues of contributing factors, which may be necessary to measure as well to provide a complete picture and determine appropriate actions to take to rectify a problem or make a change in order to improve overall health.

3.2 Privacy and Ethical Issues in Measuring Emotion

While there are certainly privacy issues surrounding the capture and use of typical personal informatics data such as location and activity level, the risk to the individual is potentially much greater when we consider capturing data regarding emotional state. One area is the ability of marketers to target potential customers at a deeply personal and more vulnerable level. The risk of mis-use of emotion data to manipulate actions seems to be greater than with other personal tracking metrics.

3.3 Goal Setting for Emotions

Another significant difference between personal informatics health tracking systems and emotion tracking systems is in the area of goal setting. If an individual wants to lose weight, for example, it is relatively easy to monitor the two primary components: input of calories and amount of exercise. If an individual wants to be happier, it is not clear that there are general quantifiable goals that can be tracked to help meet this objective. A more context-specific and personalized strategy is needed in order to support the user to achieve her/his objectives.

It is likely that the strategies necessary to achieve desired changes in emotion [1] will be more complex than those needed to change more straightforward health behaviors. Transparency in thoroughly explaining any decisions regarding recommendations would be essential to establish the level of trust that would support such major initiatives.

4 Conclusion

This paper has provided a very high-level overview of emotion tracking applications. It is not possible here to provide a thorough discussion of research linking emotion tracking and health or an in-depth description of the various technologies that support emotion tracking. Our examination of existing emotion-tracking applications provides a baseline from which to move forward in designing applications that support health through self-tracking of emotions. While there are useful features in some of these apps, such as the ability to customize the particular data that is recorded and to reach out to social networks, much more functionality is needed and is in fact possible with today's IOT technology. We have sensors that can measure biological and neurological responses and states continuously, and these can become part of future IOT emotion-management systems. Via our context-aware IOT networks we can collect data on a broad array of environmental factors that may influence stress, emotions, and the ability to respond to them to allow us to design applications that can be not only context-aware but also emotion-aware.

Additional research is needed to determine the appropriateness of goal setting in the area of emotional health, and perhaps to find other means to support individuals who are striving to change their emotional state or response. In addition, tools will be needed to support the tracking and reporting of emotion data to aid users in the appropriate interpretation of the data and to create self-learning environments where not only can users measure their emotional states, but can also determine the best individualized means to achieve positive results.

Acknowledgments. This work was partially financed by the Knowledge Foundation through the Internet of Things and People research profile.

References

1. DeSteno, D., Gross, J.J., Kubzansky, L.: Affective science and health: the importance of emotion and emotion regulation. Health Psychol. **32**(5), 474–486 (2013)
2. Fredrickson, B.L.: What Good are Positive Emotions? Rev. Gen. Psychol. **2**, 300–319 (1998)
3. Kubzansky, L.D., Park, N., Peterson, C., Vokonas, P., Sparrow, D.: Healthy psychological functioning and incident coronary heart disease: the importance of self-regulation. Arch. Gen. Psychiatry **68**, 400–408 (2011)
4. Pressman, S.D., Cohen, S.: Does positive affect influence health? Psychol. Bull. **131**, 925–971 (2005)
5. Izard, C.E.: The many meanings/aspects of emotion: definitions, functions, activation, and regulation. Emot. Rev. **2**, 363–370 (2010)
6. Barrett, L.F., Mesquita, B., Ochsner, K.N., Gross, J.J.: The experience of emotion. Ann. Rev. Psychol. **58**, 373–403 (2007)
7. Ohlin, F., Olsson, C.M., Davidsson, P.: Analyzing the design space of personal informatics: a state-of-practice based classification of existing tools. In: Antona, M., Stephanidis, C. (eds.) UAHCI 2015. LNCS, vol. 9175, pp. 85–97. Springer, Cham (2015). doi:10.1007/978-3-319-20678-3_9
8. Russell, J.A., Weiss, A., Mendelsohn, G.A.: Affect grid: a single-item scale of pleasure and arousal. J. Pers. Soc. Psychol. **57**, 493 (1989)

TEEM: A Mobile App for Technology-Enhanced Emergency Management

Massimo Canonico[1], Stefania Montani[1], and Manuel Striani[2(✉)]

[1] DISIT, Computer Science Institute,
University of Piemonte Orientale, Alessandria, Italy
{massimo.canonico,stefania.montani}@uniupo.it
[2] Computer Science Department, University of Torino, Turin, Italy
striani@di.unito.it

Abstract. In this paper we describe a mobile app for *Technology-Enhanced Emergency Management* (TEEM), designed for supporting data recording and transmission during patient transportation by ambulance. TEEM allows the travelling personnel to record the most significant patient data, and to send them to the destination center, where the specialist physician will be notified and allowed to inspect the data themselves, possibly providing immediate advice. The exploitation of TEEM also allows to maintain the transportation data over time, for medico-legal purposes, or to perform a-posteriori analyses. The app is currently under evaluation at the Neonatal Intensive Care Unit of Alessandria Children Hospital, Italy.

Keywords: Mobile app · Mobile cloud computing · Data recording · Data transmission · Emergency patient management

1 Introduction

Patients experiencing a medical emergency (e.g., stroke patients, pre-term born babies, or accident victims) are normally taken to the closest hospital structure, which might be insufficiently equipped, in terms of human or instrumental resources, to address their needs. In these situations, the patient has to be stabilized, and then carried to a larger and more suitable health care center, where specialized physicians and all necessary diagnostic/therapeutic devices are available.

During patient transportation by ambulance, a specialist physician (e.g., a neurologist) is typically not present; assistance is usually provided by paramedics and/or emergency medicine doctors. The patient is continuously monitored by means of proper devices available on the ambulance (such as ECG or blood pressure monitor). However, the monitored data, at least in Italy, are not automatically recorded. Therefore, they cannot be inspected/analyzed a posteriori. Moreover, they are not accessible in real time by the specialist physician at the destination reference center.

In this paper, we propose a mobile app for *Technology-Enhanced Emergency Management* (TEEM), specifically studied for patient transportation by ambulance.

© ICST Institute for Computer Sciences, Social Informatics and Telecommunications Engineering 2016
M.U. Ahmed et al. (Eds.): HealthyIoT 2016, LNICST 187, pp. 101–106, 2016.
DOI: 10.1007/978-3-319-51234-1_16

TEEM allows the physician or paramedic personnel to record the most significant patient data (generated by monitoring devices or directly measured), and to immediately send them to the destination center, where the specialist physician will be notified and allowed to inspect the data themselves, thus having a more complete understanding of the patient's situation already during transportation. In case of need, the physician will also be able to communicate with the ambulance personnel and supervise the management of possible critical needs in real time.

TEEM has been designed to be secure, but also extremely user friendly in its design, since the travelling personnel must not be distracted from more critical tasks (i.e., patient management).

The exploitation of TEEM will not only support real-time communication, but will also allow to record the most significant data, maintaining them for medico-legal purposes, or to perform a-posteriori intra and inter-patient analyses (e.g., for a more complete patient characterization, or for quality assessment of the medical center).

TEEM has been specifically designed for pre-term born baby transportation, but could be easily be extended to different application domains as well.

2 Technology-Enhanced Emergency Management in the Ambulance

The TEEM mobile app, in its current version, has been realized to monitor the transportation of pre-term born babies. The application domain specificities will be quickly illustrated in Sect. 2.1. Section 2.2 will then provide the details of the technical and methodological choices. Section 2.3 will illustrate the main characteristics of the client side interface, to be used by the ambulance personnel on a smartphone, and Sect. 2.4 will provide a description of the server side interface, to be used by the specialist physician at the hospital.

2.1 Pre-term Born Baby Transportation

Pre-term born babies are very often critical patients, who need intensive care. If a baby is born at an insufficiently equipped hospital, s/he has to be moved to a hospital equipped with a *Neonatal Intensive Care Unit* (NICU) [1]. Transportation may also be required if the baby, possibly already cared at the NICU, needs a specific intervention, that can be performed only at a larger or more specialized clinical center.

The clinical conditions of the baby to be transported may require ventilation assistance during the journey. Three different types of mechanical ventilations exist, each of them requiring specific parameter settings. Different transportation types must therefore be considered.

2.2 Related Work

Recently, architectures for storing and analyzing medical data in cloud computing [2] have been proposed in combination with the usage of mobile devices, which allow to send/receive data in real time without any particular equipment and/or knowledge. This new computing paradigm is called *Mobile Cloud Computing* (MCC) [3]. MCC integrates the cloud computing into the mobile environment and overcomes obstacles related to the performance (e.g., battery life, storage, and bandwidth), environment (e.g., heterogeneity, scalability, and availability), and security (e.g., reliability and privacy) discussed in mobile computing. When adopting MCC, low bandwidth issues from the mobile communication side, and security, confidentiality and integrity issues from the cloud computing side have often to be considered. Bandwidth issues have been dealt with in the approaches in [4, 5], which propose solutions to share the limited bandwidth among mobile users. As for security/integrity/confidentiality issues, a classical solution [6] consists of three main components: a mobile device, a web and storage service and a trusted third party. This third party is in charge of running a trusted crypto coprocessor which generates a *Message Authentication Code* (MAC). Thanks to the MAC, every request from the user to read/write data on cloud storage is properly authenticated and, at any time, it is possible to validate the integrity of any file, collection of files or the whole file system stored in the cloud.

2.3 System Architecture

In our system, we have adopted the MCC paradigm. To adopt MCC in our scenario, we had to address both low bandwidth issues from the mobile communication side, and security/integrity/confidentiality issues on storing medical data from the cloud computing side. To address bandwidth issues we have resorted on the already cited approaches in [4, 5], while for security/integrity/confidentiality issues, we have resorted to the three component architecture described in [6]. The overall system architecture is illustrated in Fig. 1.

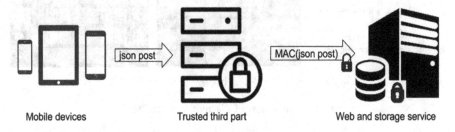

Mobile devices   Trusted third part   Web and storage service

Fig. 1. System architecture.

2.4   The TEEM App: Client Side

The TEEM app is meant to be exploited in very critical situations, where the user has higher priorities with respect to data entry. At the same time, key transportation data are extremely useful for the specialist, and of course need to be correct. Given these goals, the mobile app has been designed to be very user friendly, very clear, and essential in its graphical design.

As observed in Sect. 2.1, different types of patients may be transported: those requiring mechanical ventilation, and those who are able to breathe autonomously. In order to minimize the number of data to be inserted, and to avoid mistakes, TEEM immediately asks to select whether the patient has to be ventilated or not. In case of ventilation, the user will further set the correct ventilation type. In this way, instrumental setting data will be required only in the appropriate cases.

Overall, the parameters to be inputted have been selected by our medical collaborators, on the basis of domain knowledge.

Every data entry operation has been customized on the basis of the type of data being inputted, in order to make it as fast and simple as possible, as illustrated in Fig. 2. The figure presents three different activities of the TEEM app, that allow the user to input some data for a non-ventilated transportation.

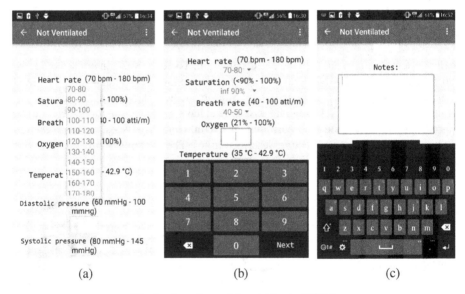

Fig. 2.   Snapshots of 3 activities in TEEM.

In Fig. 2(a), heart frequency is being inputted. In our application domain, the exact value of heart frequency is not of interest: only the range needs to be specified. To this end, a set of pre-defined ranges are shown to the user, who will just have to choose one of them without digitizing any number. Pre-defined ranges have been defined on the basis of medical knowledge as well.

In the second activity (Fig. 2(b)), oxygen saturation has to be inserted. The admissibility range (21%–100%) is reminded to the user, but s/he has then to insert a specific numeric value. To this end, a numeric keyboard is activated.

It is worth noting that consistency controls are also executed in this case, since, as observed above, transportation data always need to be correct. If the digitized number is outside the admissibility range, an error message will appear, in order to allow the user to introduce the correct value.

Finally, in the third case (Fig. 2(c)), additional textual notes can be inserted. In this case, an alpha-numeric keyboard with auto-completion is activated.

When data have been sent to the server, the user is notified by a toast message, i.e., a notification message that shows for a few seconds and then fades away.

2.5 Server Side

The data inputted by the user through the mobile app interface are then serialized as a JSON string, which is posted to the server (see Fig. 1). At the server side, data have to be de-serialized, stored in a database, and shown to the user through a web interface.

The web page is automatically refreshed every five seconds, in order to always show the most recent data during transportation. Indeed, an updated measurement can be send several times during the journey.

Data are stored in a database, which maintains all the measured information, for medico-legal purpose, and constitutes an important knowledge source for the hospital. Indeed, historical data can also be queried, and shown to the user through the web interface, for further investigation, or for comparison with different patient cases.

3   Conclusions and Future Work

In this paper we have described TEEM, a mobile app studied to support data communication during patient transportation by ambulance. TEEM allows the ambulance personnel to insert the most significant patient monitoring data, and immediately send them to the destination center, thus substituting the extremely incomplete paper log that is currently deployed. TEEM has been designed to be user-friendly, but also to guarantee data entry correctness. Interestingly, we are not aware of any other similar approach in the field of emergency patient transportation.

TEEM is currently being made available to the personnel of the NICU of Alessandria Children Hospital, Italy. The NICU has 7 beds, and usually performs more than 80 transportations a year. After a testing period, TEEM will be revised/enhanced as needed, and then made available for routine adoption.

In parallel, we are working at the implementation of a second mobile app, directly interfaced to the monitoring devices of the ambulance. This second app is meant to automatically send to the hospital server all the data measured by the devices, in real time. It will complement TEEM (which will still be used to insert non-instrumental data), and will allow the specialist physician to receive a significant amount of information during transportation. This will enable her/him to have a very clear picture of the patient's situation as soon as s/he arrives at the hospital, and thus to immediately start the proper treatment, without having to re-asses the patient condition, as it currently happens.

Acknowledgments. We acknowledge Dr. D. Gazzolo and Dr. M.C. Strozzi for providing their knowledge about pre-term neonatal care, and about the specifics of the service we have designed. This research is original and has a financial support of the University of Piemonte Orientale.

References

1. http://apps.who.int/iris/bitstream/10665/183037/1/9789241508988_eng.pdf. Last Accessed 8 Sept 2016
2. Li, M., et al.: Scalable and secure sharing of personal health records in cloud computing using attribute-based encryption. IEEE Trans. Parallel Distrub. Syst. **24**(1), 131–143 (2013)
3. Fernando, N., Loke, N.W., Rahayu, W.: Mobile cloud computing: a survey. Future Gener. Comput. Syst. **29**(2), 84–106 (2013)
4. Jin, X., Kwok, Y.K.: Cloud assisted P2P media streaming for bandwidth constrained mobile subscribers. In: Proceedings of the 16th IEEE International Conference on Parallel and Distributed Systems (ICPADS) (2011)
5. Misra, S., Das, S., Khatua, M., Obaidat, M.S.: QoS-guaranteed bandwidth shifting and redistribution in mobile cloud environment. Trans. Cloud Comput. **2**(2), 181–193 (2014)
6. Zhou, Z., Huang, D.: Efficient and secure data storage operations for mobile cloud computing. In: Proceedings of the 8th International Conference on Network and Service Management (2013)

Perception of Delay in Computer Input Devices Establishing a Baseline for Signal Processing of Motion Sensor Systems

Jiaying Du[1,2(✉)], Daniel Kade[1,2], Christer Gerdtman[2], Rikard Lindell[1], Oguzhan Özcan[3], and Maria Lindén[1]

[1] School of Innovation, Design and Engineering, Mälardalen University, Högskoleplan 1, 72123 Västerås, Sweden
jiaying.du@mdh.se

[2] Motion Control i Västerås AB, Ängsgärdsgatan 10, 72130 Västerås, Sweden

[3] Arçelik Research Center for Creative Industries, Koç University, Rumelifeneri, 34450 Sarıyer, İstanbul, Turkey

Abstract. New computer input devices in healthcare applications using small embedded sensors need firmware filters to run smoothly and to provide a better user experience. Therefore, it has to be investigated how much delay can be tolerated for signal processing before the users perceive a delay when using a computer input device. This paper is aimed to find out a threshold of unperceived delay by performing user tests with 25 participants. A communication retarder was used to create delays from 0 to 100 ms between a receiving computer and three different USB-connected computer input devices. A wired mouse, a wifi mouse and a head-mounted mouse were used as input devices. The results of the user tests show that delays up to 50 ms could be tolerated and are not perceived as delay, or depending on the used device still perceived as acceptable.

Keywords: Computer mouse · Delay · Embedded systems · Healthcare · Perception · USB

1 Introduction

Developing firmware without hindering users to perform tasks in their ability is of importance for small wearable sensor systems, especially in healthcare applications. Early developed gyroscope based computer head mice [1] and similar systems need filtering and smoothing of sensor data to work properly, as sensors used in wearable systems are appreciated to be small, light, cheap and usually have the drawbacks of high sensitivity to environmental disturbances [2,3]. Signal processing and its resulting delay are main factors on system performance.

In the previous research, system latency has already been seen as a primary concern in providing real-time interaction for human-computer interfaces [4]. The effect of delay in the quality of video and voice communication [5], in video

© ICST Institute for Computer Sciences, Social Informatics and Telecommunications Engineering 2016
M.U. Ahmed et al. (Eds.): HealthyIoT 2016, LNICST 187, pp. 107–112, 2016.
DOI: 10.1007/978-3-319-51234-1_17

streaming [6], between visual information and tactile information [7], in haptic environments [8] have been analyzed. Unnoticeable delay of approximately 150 ms for keyboard interactions and up to 195 ms for mouse interactions were found by detecting changes in a graphical user interface [9].

Moreover, to investigate how long calculations and filters can run in the firmware of an embedded device, studies have been conducted to find out the user perception of unperceived, acceptable, disturbing and unacceptable delays. Previously, research has been performed to investigate the first indicator on how delay between 0 and 500 ms was perceived by users. With a common computer mouse, delays up to 150 ms have been demonstrated as acceptable delay, while delays over 300 ms were regarded as unacceptable and delays between 150 ms and 300 ms were perceived by users as disturbing [10]. The results provided a baseline on the limit of acceptable delay for data processing in microprocessors, embedded systems or other similar applications. However, more thoroughly studies are needed to investigate the interval below 100 ms delay and to consider the effect of using different USB input devices.

The aim of this paper was to better understand the user's perception of delay when using different input computer devices and to find out a more precise baseline allowing to set a limit for signal processing in small embedded sensor systems. Therefore, we performed user tests with 25 participants who tested three different computer input devices with settings of 0 ms, 25 ms, 50 ms, 75 ms and 100 ms of delay in alternating order for each input device. This paper focuses on (1) How much delay can be set until users perceive the delay? (2) What is the difference when using different computer input devices with divergent sensitivity? (3) Is there a difference between interaction methods, such as hand movement or head movement?

2   Research Approach

To change the values of delay in a controlled way, the communication retarder as described in [10] was used to generate delays. Software was developed to perform a click task for users and to collect user data. A wired computer mouse with USB cable, an USB wifi mouse and a head-mounted mouse called MultiPos were connected to the communication retarder called USB-delay. An overview of the test setup can be seen in Fig. 1.

To collect user feedback and data for evaluations and investigations, user tests were performed during 2 days with 25 persons, 22 male and 3 female participants, from the age of 24 to 52 with an average age of 34.7. All participants were daily computer users without mobility impairment. Most users (22/25) were using a computer mouse daily. The other 3 users were using a trackpad for daily uses. Most users had never used a head-mounted mouse before. Only one user tested a head movement controlled game.

The hardware for our tests, shown in Fig. 1, consisted of a gaming laptop (MSI MS-16GF) with Windows 10, an in-house developed communication retarder (USB-delay device), a gaming mousepad (Logitech G240), a wired gaming mouse

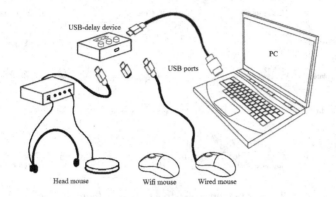

Fig. 1. System overview.

(Logitech M500), a wifi mouse (Packard Bell MORFEOUO) and a MEMS gyroscope based head-mounted computer mouse (MultiPos).

At the beginning of each test, the testers were informed about the purpose of the study, their tasks and the procedure. Each user tested three different devices for 5 rounds with 5 different delay values. The users' task was to click on 4 emerging images on the screen with unknown but fixed locations in each round. As done in the previous research, the order was chosen to start with a neutral setting of 0 ms, giving the testers a baseline of the mouse sensitivity and time to adapt to the tests [10]. Then the delay between higher and lower settings was alternated. In order to gather information about the users' experiences, a questionnaire was required to be answered. The perceived level of delay that the user perceived was asked in the form of choosing a score between four perceived levels: (1) 'unacceptable', (2) 'disturbing', (3) 'acceptable' and (4) 'no delay perceived'. After every round the users rated their experience with the device at the set delay value. Additionally, data was collected on how long it took the users to click on the emerging images and if users were able to click the images through our developed software. The collected data and the feedback from the users was then analysed with the help of MATLAB.

3   Results and Discussion

The results of our evaluations and the user feedbacks are described statistically in Fig. 2. Here, the amount of feedback is presented by different sized red points in combination with a number, reflecting the users' questionnaire choices. The blue curve connects the majority levels and shows the main trend of the perceived results. For the wired mouse the delay of 50 ms can be seen as the threshold value between 'no delay perceived' and 'acceptable'. In other words, the delays smaller than 50 ms were not perceived by the users using the wired mouse. The tests and evaluation also show that the delay perception of the users is affected by the sensitivity of the USB devices. With a low sensitivity wifi mouse,

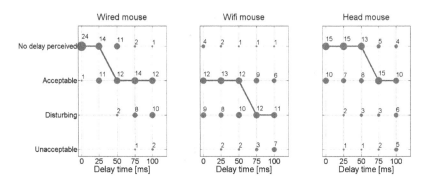

Fig. 2. User perceived feedback. (Color figure online)

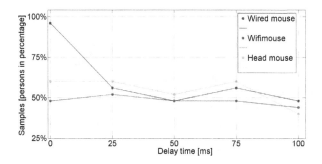

Fig. 3. Majority distribution. (Color figure online)

50 ms of delay can still be seen as threshold value, but scored a lower perception rating between 'acceptable' and 'disturbing'. The head-mounted mouse has more sensitivity because of a more precise MEMS gyroscope. Here, more users did not perceive delays up to 50 ms in comparison to the other two devices.

Figure 3 presents the majority distribution of the three different devices used in this research. The blue curve depicts the results of the wired computer mouse, while the red one presents for the wifi mouse and the green curve is for the head-mounted mouse. Almost 100% of the users (24/25) gave the same feedback for the delay of 0 ms with the wired mouse. In the continuation of the comparison, more than 50% of the users had similar opinions for the delays of 25 ms, 50 ms, 75 ms and 100 ms, respectively. For the head-mounted mouse, except the delay of 100 ms, around 60% of the users showed similar perceptions with the delays of 0 ms, 25 ms, 50 ms and 75 ms. For the wifi mouse, around 50% of the users perceived similar results with all five delay values. In general, users showed the most different perceptions with the wifi mouse.

The elapsed time for clicking the four images in each round was recorded in our software. The data was averaged by images and users. The average clicking time of the different delays from 0 ms to 100 ms is 1.56 s with the wired mouse, 1.87 s with the wifi mouse and 2.22 s with the head-mounted mouse. The trends

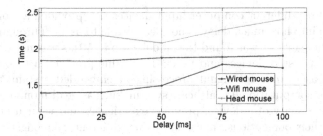

Fig. 4. Elapsed time. (Color figure online)

of elapsed time for the three different devices are depicted in Fig. 4. The blue curve presents the results of the wired mouse, the red curve is for the wifi mouse and the green curve shows the results for the head-mounted device. The elapsed time to click on the images is increasing as the delay increases. As shown with the red curve, the users needed more time to click on the images with larger delays. The green curve shows that it takes more time to click on the images with the head-mounted mouse. Less elapsed time with the delay of 50 ms reflects that the users might have adapted to the movements after the first round. However, they still spend more time as the delay increases afterwards.

Table 1. Overview of missed images during the tests.

Delay (ms)	0	25	50	75	100	Sum
Mouse	-	1	1	2	-	4
Wifi mouse	2	5	2	3	3	15
Head mouse	8	19	4	21	24	76
Sum	10	25	7	26	27	95

During the tests 1500 images were clickable in total (25 users × 3 devices/ user × 5 rounds/device × 4 images/round). The images disappeared after 3 s in case a user could not click on it. Totally 95 missed images were recorded during the test, 22 for first appearing image, 22 for the second image, 33 for the third image and 18 for the fourth image. Table 1 shows the number of missed images with different delay values and devices. As shown in Fig. 4 and Table 1, generally it took users the most time and the most misses happened when using the head-mounted mouse, while the least time and misses happened when using the wired mouse. In general, we can say that the greater the delay is, the more time to click on the images was needed and the more misses happened.

4   Conclusion

A previous study has shown the effects of USB-delay on a broad delay range from 0 ms to 500 ms [10]. In this paper, we have further investigated the effects of delay in three different computer input devices and provided a more detailed investigation into how much delay is not perceivable to users. Through user tests with 25 participants, it was found that a delay up to 50 ms was not perceived as delay for most tested devices and users. This value provided a threshold value that we see as a limit for signal processing in embedded systems, especially body-worn or computational healthcare systems such as head-mounted computer mice. The sensitivity of a device, previous experiences and what users are used to, affected their perceptions. These individual differences amongst users could for example be seen with a simple, less sensitive wifi mouse, as users rated their experience with lower scores. Using an uncommon and unknown technology of a MEMS gyroscope based head-mounted computer mouse, users needed more time to click on appearing images as users needed to move their heads in comparison to the hand-controlled mice. Nonetheless, the perceived results were even better with a delay of 50 ms or less, in comparison to computer mice due to the high sensitivity of the MEMS gyroscope.

References

1. Gerdtman, C., Bäcklund, Y., Lindén, M.: A gyro sensor based computer mouse with a USB interface: a technical aid for motor-disabled people technology and disability. Technol. Disabil. **24**(2), 117–127 (2012)
2. Du, J., Gerdtman, C., Lindén, M.: Signal processing algorithms for temperature drift in a MEMS-gyro-based head mouse. In: 21st International Conference on Systems, Signals and Image Processing, pp. 123–126. IEEE Press (2014)
3. Du, J., Gerdtman, C., Lindén, M.: Noise reduction for a MEMS-gyroscope-based head mouse. In: 12th International Conference on Wearable Micro and Nano Technologies for Personalized Health, pp. 98–104. IOS Press (2015)
4. Carlson, J., Han, R., Lao, S., Narayan, C., Sanghani, S.: Rapid prototyping of mobile input devices using wireless sensor nodes. In: 5th IEEE Workshop on Mobile Computing Systems and Applications, pp. 21–29. IEEE Press (2003)
5. Kurita, T., Iai, S., Kitawaki, N.: Assessing the effects of transmission delay - interaction of speech and video. In: 14th International Symposium: Human Factors in Telecommunications Proceedings, pp. 111–121 (1993)
6. Bhamidipati, V.D., Kilari, S.: Effect of Delay/Delay Variable on QoE in Video Streaming. Master thesis, School of Computing at Blekinge Institute of Technology (2010)
7. Miyasato, T., Noma, H., Kishino, F.: Subjective evaluation of perception of delay time between visual information and tactile information. IEICE Trans. Fundam. Electron. Commun. Comput. Sci. **79**(5), 655–657 (1996)
8. Rank, M., Shi, Z., Müller, H.J., Hirche, S.: Perception of delay in haptic telepresence systems. Presence **19**(5), 389–399 (2010)
9. Dabrowski, J.R., Munson, E.V.: Is 100 milliseconds too fast? In: CHI 2001 Extended Abstracts on Human Factors in Computing Systems, pp. 317–318 (2001)
10. Du, J., Kade, D., Gerdtman, C., Özcan, O., Lindén, M.: The effects of perceived USB delay for sensor and embedded system development. In: Proceedings of the 38th Annual International Conference of the IEEE Engineering in Medicine and Biology Society, pp. 2492–2495. IEEE Press (2016)

Telemetry System for Diagnosis of Asthma and Chronical Obstructive Pulmonary Disease (COPD)

Eldar Granulo[1], Lejla Bećar[2], Lejla Gurbeta[3,4],
and Almir Badnjević[1,3,4(✉)]

[1] Faculty of Electrical Engineering, University of Sarajevo,
Sarajevo, Bosnia and Herzegovina
egranulo2@etf.unsa.ba
[2] Faculty of Medicine, University of Sarajevo,
Sarajevo, Bosnia and Herzegovina
becar.lejla@gmail.com
[3] Verlab Ltd., Sarajevo, Bosnia and Herzegovina
almir.badnjevic@verlab.ba
[4] International Burch University, Ilidža, Bosnia and Herzegovina
gurbeta.lejla@ibu.edu.ba

Abstract. For people who live in rural or remote areas, or have a limited possibility of movement, disease is diagnosed late in the course, which unfortunately often results in death. In order to increase awareness among people and to reduce mortality rates, telemetry systems play a very important role. This paper presents the telemetry system for diagnosis of Asthma and COPD (COPD - Chronic obstructive pulmonary disease, a type of obstructive lung disease characterized by long-term poor airflow). Developed telemetry system is implemented using Android, Java, MATLAB and PHP technologies. Classification of respiratory diseases is implemented in our previous papers. During the six months' period telemetry system was tested on 541 subjects, where 324 were classified as asthmatics or COPD while 217 were classified as healthy subjects. Implemented system uses a spirometer connected via Bluetooth with a mobile phone application for sending data to the server where is installed Expert System for classification of Asthma and COPD. After the classification process Expert System is sending a diagnosis to the patient via e-mail.

Keywords: Telemetry · Expert System · Disease · Classification · Asthma · COPD

1 Introduction

The constant development of information - communication technologies (ICT) [1] results in increased use of these technologies in everyday medical practice and change the way of patient care. The combination of intelligent computer systems and mobile applications allow more involvement of patients in the care of their own health through interactive exchange of information with trained medical staff. In Europe in the last

© ICST Institute for Computer Sciences, Social Informatics and Telecommunications Engineering 2016
M.U. Ahmed et al. (Eds.): HealthyIoT 2016, LNICST 187, pp. 113–118, 2016.
DOI: 10.1007/978-3-319-51234-1_18

15 years (2000–2015) the number of Internet users increased for 454.2%, and statistics show that approximately 70.5% of the population in Europe has Internet access [2]. Cisco predicts that by the end of 2016 there will be 10 billion mobile devices worldwide in use [3]. Surveys carried out in European hospitals in the period 2012–2013 year [4] and general practitioners (2013) [5] showed that 9% of hospitals offer patients the possibility of using Internet applications in monitoring their health status. Studies in the United States in 2012, showed that 39% of the surveyed doctors use Internet and Web applications to communicate with patients, an increase of 8% as compared to [6]. In study published by Hardinge et al. [7] patients identified no difficulties in using the proposed Internet application and were able to use all implemented functions.

According to the World Health Organization (WHO), there are around 600 million patients with COPD and 344 million patients with asthma today in the world, which is double than diabetics and it is predicted to 2020, that COPD will become the world's third biggest cause of mortality [8], and thus the main growing public health problem. In recent years, several applications have been proposed to improve and ease the diagnosis of these diseases. Badnjevic et al. in their papers developed Expert System for diagnosis of respiratory diseases such as asthma and COPD based on combination of fuzzy rules and artificial neural network [9]. In papers [10, 11] they presented a system for diagnosis of asthma based just on fuzzy rules or developed artificial neural network, where they showed an importance of usage of Expert systems in healthcare institutions. In all mentioned papers they used spirometry (SPIR)[1] and/or Impulse Oscillometry (IOS) as input measuring parameters. Expert System results are convenient to read and analyze as they are presented in simple forms of texts and figures [12, 13]. The benefits of telemedicine have been shown in other papers [15], which has found that the application of the same procedure to each spirometry examination data and its central processing ensures that all the necessary procedures and checks are carried out with full compliance to the standards of the medical profession [16].

2 Methodology – Telemetry System

The developed telemetry system consists of mobile application and Expert System. Telemetry application will interact with the patient through user interface in several steps. In first step, SPIR test is conducted. Then, measured parameters are stored in mobile phone in .pdf format. In step 3, symptoms of disease for patients are indicated in mobile application. After that, measurement results and symptoms indication are transferred to server. Input vector for Expert System is formed in step 5. After that classification is performed and in final step test results are sent to user's mobile phone. Detailed system architecture and data flow is presented in Fig. 1. Developed telemetry system is implemented using a combination of technologies which include Android, Java, Matlab and PHP. Android and Java are used for implementing a simple mobile application that allows the user to upload the results of a conducted measurements.

---

[1] SPIR - Spirometry (meaning the measuring of breath) is the most common of the pulmonary function tests (PFTs), measuring lung function, specifically the amount (volume) and/or speed (flow) of air that can be inhaled and exhaled.

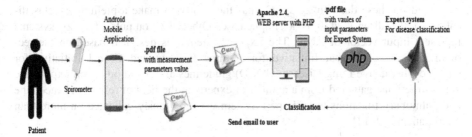

Fig. 1. Architecture of implemented telemetry system.

Expert System for classification of respiratory disease is implemented in Matlab. PHP programming language is used to parse the uploaded .pdf files and to call Matlab functions in the background. The input data of developed telemetry system are spirometry (SPIR) test results and symptoms of disease. For obtaining measurement result spirometers with communication module (Bluetooth communication module is used in this paper) must be used in order to get measurement results on used mobile phone. To obtain usable measurement results, examination protocol must be followed. To ensure that measured data are in accordance to Expert System input parameters format, error check is implemented, in the sense that the document with measurement results contains all necessary data for classification. If the check is successful, the file is wrapped in an HTTP POST request and sent to address of the server. Expert System is located on server. In this study, Apache 2.4 Server is used. Once, the input data are given to Expert System classification based on measurement results and symptoms is conducted and the results of classification performed by Expert System are sent to user by email.

A. Expert System

Expert System for classification of respiratory disease consists of Artificial Neural Network (ANN) and Fuzzy rules. The possible outputs of classification are: Normal condition, Asthma, COPD and Additional testing needed on the Pulmonary Clinic. Architecture of Expert System is presented in Fig. 2 [9]. The input data for the implemented fuzzy rules are values obtained by conducting spirometry (SPIR) test.

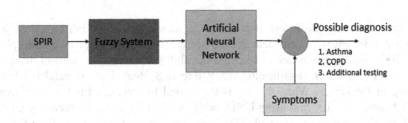

Fig. 2. Architecture of Expert System.

116   E. Granulo et al.

Based on these data, fuzzy system has the ability to make a preliminary classification of the disease, if it is a simple case. Otherwise, outputs of fuzzy systems represent input vector of ANN. The Expert System was designed based on the recommendations of Global Initiative for Asthma (GINA) and Global Initiative for Chronic Obstructive Lung Disease (GOLD) guidelines and based on expert experience and instructions, gathered from a number of experts in the field of respiratory medicine and pulmonary functions tests. Expert System was previously validated on more than 1000 patients [9–14].

B. Mobile application
The mobile application is developed for the Android operating system and it was implemented in Java using Android Studio 2.0 integrated development environment. The structure is relatively simple, which opens it to development for different mobile operating systems in the future. An activity diagram representing the application flow is shown in Fig. 3.

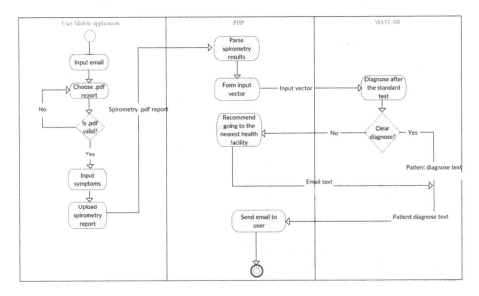

Fig. 3. Application activity diagram

After conducting SPIR test, user stores the measured data in .pdf format on used mobile phone. Measurement data are transferred from spirometer to mobile phone using Bluetooth communication. User has the ability to insert symptoms of disease in order to ensure better classification using Expert System. Data is validated before sending to the server. When the file is transferred to server, a PHP script activates which handles the file, first using UNIX pdf to text utility with a preserve layout flag, which writes the data to a text file. The script then loads the content of the file as a string, then using regular expressions, parses the measurements and forms an input vector for the Expert System. The Expert System gives an assessment, as is shown in Fig. 1. Since PHP cannot interact directly with Matlab, the results are written to console output and read by PHP. These results, along with the symptoms and patient data form a report which is written to an email and sent to the user. The user receives a confirmation email that his report was successfully uploaded.

3 Results

During the design of the application, usability in accordance with ISO 9126 software quality model was followed. The developed application has relatively straightforward design, icons and information assistance. The time needed for installation and setup is minimum. The main function is sending an email with measurement data and symptoms indication from patient in order to establish quick diagnosis of possible respiratory disease in real time in remote areas. The entire process that takes part on the server side, takes on average ten seconds. When compared to the time needed to obtain the necessary documents to visit a doctor, the application allows the user to quickly identify his condition, or directs him to a physician to conduct more tests. To validate the integrated software suite, reports of 541 patients who have previously visited departments for lungs diseases have been used. There were 25 patients with diagnosed COPD, 72 patients with asthma and 217 patients treated as a healthy control group.

4 Conclusion

One of the greatest challenges in rural healthcare system is assuring that professional medical presence is available when and where it is needed. This is difficult for remote rural healthcare institutions because they are often intractable for those medical professionals or those institutions cannot afford or retain these specialty providers. In today's healthcare systems telemedicine is reflected through synchronized data exchange and the advantage of telemedicine/biotelemetry is that recordings of signals of patients are done under the standard conditions, so that stress does not create artifacts that distort the typical form of the signal and subsequent diagnosis on the basis of the recorded signal is more accurate since they are used more realistic signals.

The developed telemetry system described in this paper enables patients living in remote areas, or patients with limited ability of movement to establish a diagnosis based on results of spirometry obtained from a simple to use spirometer. This enables better self-management for patients since they are able to track their health condition and if needed get adequate professional care.

References

1. Beniger, J.R.: The Control Revolution: Technological and Economic Origins of the Information Society. Harvard University Press, Cambridge (1986)
2. Internet World Statistics. www.Internetworldstats.com/stats.com
3. International Telecommunication Union (ITU): Internet users per 100 inhabitants 1997 to 2007. ICT Data and Statistics (IDS)

118   E. Granulo et al.

4. European Hospital Survey - Benchmarking Deployment of eHealth services, 2012–2013
5. Benchmarking Deployment of eHealth among General Practitioners (2013)
6. American EHR Partners: "Mobile Usage in the Medical Space 2013" and "Tablet Usage by Physicians 2013"
7. Hardinge, M., Rutter, H., Velardo, C., Ahmar, S.S., Williams, V., Tarassenko, L., Farmer, A.: Using a mobile health application to support self-management in chronic obstructive pulmonary disease: a six-month cohort study. BMC Med. Inform. Decis. Making 15(1), 1 (2015)
8. Murray, C.J., Lopez, A.D.: Alternative projections of mortality and disability cause 1990–2020: Global Burden of Disease Study. Lancet 349, 1498–1504 (1997)
9. Badnjevic, A., Gurbeta, L., Cifrek, M., Marjanovic, D.: Diagnostic of asthma using fuzzy rules implemented in accordance with international guidelines and physicians experience. In: IEEE 39th International Convention on Information and Communication Technology, Electronics and Microelectronics (MIPRO), Opatija, Croatia, 30 May to 03 June 2016
10. Badnjevic, A., Gurbeta, L., Cifrek, M., Marjanovic, D.: Classification of asthma using artificial neural network. In: IEEE 39th International Convention on Information and Communication Technology, Electronics and Microelectronics (MIPRO), Opatija, Croatia, 30 May to 03 June 2016
11. Badnjevic, A., Cifrek, M., Koruga, D.: Integrated software suite for diagnosis of respiratory diseases. In: IEEE International Conference on Computer as Tool (EUROCON), Zagreb, Croatia, pp. 564–568, 01–04 July 2013
12. Badnjevic, A., Cifrek, M., Koruga, D.: Classification of Chronic Obstructive Pulmonary Disease (COPD) using integrated software suite. In: IFMBE XIII Mediterranean Conference on Medical and Biological Engineering and Computing (MEDICON), pp. 25–28, September 2013
13. Badnjevic, A., Cifrek, M., Koruga, D., Osmankovic, D.: Neuro-fuzzy classification of asthma and chronic obstructive pulmonary disease. BMC Med. Inform. Decis. Making J. 15 (Suppl 3), S1 (2015)
14. Badnjevic, A., Cifrek, M.: Classification of asthma utilizing integrated software suite. In: 6th European Conference of the International Federation for Medical and Biological Engineering (MBEC), Dubrovnik, Croatia, pp. 07–11, September 2014
15. Burgos, F., Disdier, C., de Santamaria, E.L., Galdiz, B., Roger, N., Rivera, M.L., Hervàs, R., Durán-Tauleria, E., Garcia-Aymerich, J., Roca, J.: Telemedicine enhances quality of forced spirometry in primary care. Eur. Respir. J. 39(6), 1313–1318 (2012)
16. Soriano, J.B., Ancochea, J., Miravitlles, M.: Recent trends in COPD prevalence in Spain: a repeated cross-sectional survey 1997–2007. Eur. Respir. J. 36, 758–765 (2010)

Remotely Supporting Patients with Obstructive Sleep Apnea at Home

Xavier Rafael-Palou$^{(\boxtimes)}$, Alexander Steblin, and Eloisa Vargiu

eHealth Unit, EURECAT, Barcelona, Spain
{xavier.rafael,alexander.steblin,eloisa.vargiu}@eurecat.org
http://www.eurecat.org

Abstract. People suffering Obstructive Sleep Apnea are normally treated by using a device that provides continuous positive airway pressure. Currently solutions do not rely on any remote assistance and data gathered from that device are accessible to clinicians only when the patient goes to the annual visit. In this paper, we propose an IoT-based system that sends data to the cloud where are analyzed to support patients with Obstructive Sleep Apnea giving also a suitable feedback to lung specialists. The work is part of the Spanish project myOSA. Clinical trials with patients from the Hospital Arnau i Vilanova in Lleida (Spain) started on July 2016 and will last 6 months.

Keywords: Telemonitoring · Decision support systems · Internet of Things · eHealth · Obstructive Sleep Apnea · CPAP

1 Introduction

In the last decade, the Internet of Things (IoT) paradigm rapidly grew up gaining ground in the scenario of modern wireless telecommunications [1]. Its basic idea is the pervasive presence of a variety of things or objects (e.g., tags, sensors, actuators, smartphones, everyday objects) that are able to interact with each other and cooperate with their neighbors to reach common goals. Depending on the real-world scenario, different solutions to analyse data gathered from *things* may be applied. In case of patients' involvement, self-management tools [2], decision support systems [7], and recommender systems [4] may work with data from *things* to give support to the patients with the main goal of providing empowerment.

In this paper, we focus on eHealth and propose an IoT-based monitoring system aimed at giving automatic remote support to patients suffering Obstructive Sleep Apnea (OSA) [5], as well as a suitable feedback to lung specialists. In the literature, some work focused on monitoring patients with OSA relying on IoT has been proposed [3,6]. Our approach differs in monitoring patients to improve their adherence to the prescribed therapy. Moreover, as a secondary goal, the system also provides lung specialists with relevant monitoring information to enable a better patients' follow-up.

© ICST Institute for Computer Sciences, Social Informatics and Telecommunications Engineering 2016
M.U. Ahmed et al. (Eds.): HealthyIoT 2016, LNICST 187, pp. 119–124, 2016.
DOI: 10.1007/978-3-319-51234-1_19

2 The Proposed Solution

Currently in Spain, after a visit with a lung specialist, patients suffering OSA are treated with a continuous positive airway pressure (CPAP) machine at their home. CPAP providers guide patients on how to use the device properly and prescribe them to use the machine at least 4 h daily in order to benefit the therapy. From that moment on, the adopted medical protocol states the following visit with the specialist after 6 months and then once a year. Unfortunately, this extended period of time results in patients not following the recommended prescription and even abandoning the therapy. In fact, it may happen that, during a visit, they discover that the patients is using the CPAP less that 4 h or s/he is not using it at all. To improve patients compliance and better follow-up, we propose a solution that, connecting the CPAP with Internet and providing patients with an app in their smartphone, gives support to both patients and lung specialists. In fact, in so doing, CPAP automatically sends the collected data to the cloud where are analysed and sent back to the user through the app.

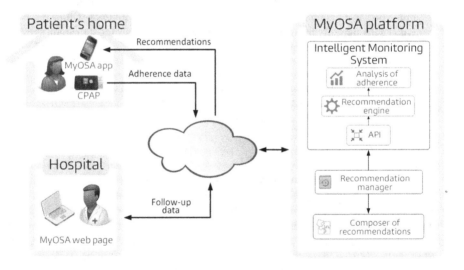

Fig. 1. Main components of the IoT-based system.

Figure 1 shows the high-level architecture of the system with its main components: *Patient's home*, *Hospital*, and *MyOSA platform*. At the *Patient's home* two devices are provided: the CPAP machine connected to Internet and a smartphone with the installed app. At the *Hospital*, lung specialists are provided with a web application that summarizes relevant information and it is aimed also to give a support in medical decisions[1]. Finally, the *MyOSA platform* is installed in the cloud and connects all the devices for data exchanging.

---

[1] The corresponding decision support system is out of the scope of this chapter.

The core of the *MyOSA platform* is the *Intelligent Monitoring System (myOSA IM)* that is composed of a set of intelligent algorithms aimed at identify the adherence level to the therapy by a given patient (*Analysis of adherence* in the Fig. 1). It includes also the *Recommendation engine* aimed at working with that adherence level to give to the *Composer of Recommendations* the list of cases that will be used to build the recommendations. The *Composer of recommendations* receives as input the cases from the *Recommendation engine* and composes the corresponding recommendations. Daily, the *Recommendation manager* receives the new monitoring data from the CPAP and puts in communication the *Composer of Recommendations* with the *Recommendation engine*, by means of the *API*, in order to get the appropriate recommendations. After that, the *Recommendation manager* sends those recommendations to the patient's app.

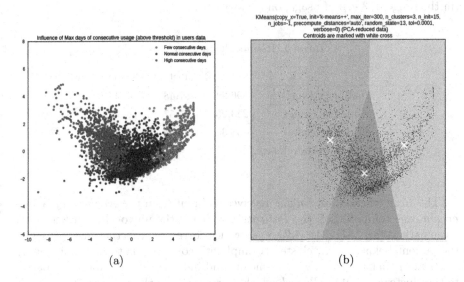

(a)   (b)

Fig. 2. PCA and K-means clustering with k = 3. (Color figure online)

The *Analysis of adherence* module is aimed at detecting the current user adherence degree to CPAP therapy given a set of monitoring data. This module wraps up a predictive model based on unsupervised learning techniques. To build this model we used data from 4207 patients (980 women) using CPAP in the Spanish area. Each patient has her/his own profile composed of basic information (e.g., age, sex, marital status), as well as a set of extra features to provide a better description of the daily CPAP usage (e.g. number of minutes of usage per day, maximum number of consecutive days using the CPAP). Once the dataset was cleaned up, the most relevant features were extracted by means of a principal component analysis (PCA) on the normalized data. The first 2 components of the PCA achieved a 0.72 of explained variance ratio. This positive result allowed to suitably visualize the amount of data with only 2 dimensions. As an example, please consider Fig. 2-a where we have projected the whole amount of data on the 2 PCA dimensions highlighting in different colors users with few, normal and high consecutive usage of the CPAP machine. After feature reduction, k-means has been used to divide patients in suitable clusters. K-means models were built using different numbers of k and the corresponding results compared by using the silhouette metric. The best results were achieved with $k = 3$ obtaining a score of 0.31. With $k = 4$, $k = 5$ and $k = 10$ scores of 0.28, 0.25 and 0.23 were obtained, respectively. Figure 2-b shows the output of the adopted clustering technique, with $k = 3$. Once the best model was selected a post processing analysis was conducted to map the resulting clusters with adherence profiles. Table 1 summarizes the results for each cluster. According to the results, Cluster0 was assigned to "Compliant" (more than 4 h of usage, on average), Cluster1 to "No-compliant" (less than 3 h of usage, on average), and Cluster2 to "Regular" (in the range of 3–4 h of usage, on average).

Table 1. Results cluster centroids.

	Cluster0	Cluster1	Cluster2
MaxUsage (min.)	596.24	357.48	546.59
MinUsage (min.)	223.25	1.57	18.32
AvgUsage (min.)	458.35	198.79	328.42
NumDaysAboveUsage	0.97	0.17	0.77

The *Recommendation Engine* receives as input from the *Analysis of Adherence* a case composed of: the *PatientID*, which is the univocal identifier of the given patient (e.g., M1234); *Adherence*, which corresponds to the cluster to which the patient belongs (e.g., cluster "Compliant" corresponds to high adherence); *Probability* that is given by the k-means and indicates the reliability to belong to the cluster (e.g., 0.8); *Period*, which corresponds to the number of monitored days that have been analyzed (e.g., weekly); *Gradient*, which is the trend corresponding to the evolution of the adherence (e.g., negative); and *Evolution* that is the number of hours corresponding to the change in the adherence. With this information the *Recommendation Engine* builds a case by relying on a rule-based approach defined according to the expertise of lung specialists.

3   Current Implementation

The proposed IoT-based myOSA IM is part of the Spanish project myOSA. CPAP users in Catalonia have been involved in experimentation. The trials just started and a total of 50 patients will participate in the study.

Once a patient enters the program, s/he is provided with a CPAP to be installed at home and an app to be installed in her/his smartphone. In particular,

Table 2. Example of recommendations.

Period biweekly		Period quarterly		Recommendation
Adherence	Gradient	Adherence	Gradient	
C	↑	–	–	Keep it up but remember to be consistent Remember that sleep well is very necessary
NC	↓	–	–	You are not following the guidelines of your doctor, you must be constant Do not get discouraged and ask for help if you need it!
NC	↓	R	↓	It has worsened the use of CPAP lately It is very important to be consistent Please contact us if you have questions!
C	↑	NC	↑	You are using more CPAP during the last two weeks, keep it up Your body will appreciate it

we use the device Airsense 10 AutoSet by RESMED[2] that includes the hardware needed for storing and transmitting the data. Once a day, the CPAP sends data to the cloud where are stored and analyzed to identify the level of adherence (i.e., the cluster) the patient belongs to. Depending on the adherence (i.e., the clusters), different recommendations are sent. Three kinds of recommendations have been identified: awards, feedback, and alerts. *Awards* are given to outstanding patients when they considerably comply with the adherence. Moreover, awards are given to empower the patient when they move from an adherence level to a higher one (e.g., from regular to compliant). *Feedback* is given anytime patients need to receive some specific recommendation to improve the use of the CPAP or to be encouraged to use it more. *Alerts* are sent when the patient belongs to the no-compliant cluster and needs to be supported. Alerts may also be sent when a patient moves from an adherence level to a lower one (e.g., from regular to no-compliant). Table 2 shows an example of recommendations with the corresponding adherence level (C for Compliant, NC for No-Compliant, and R for Regular) and the gradient (↑ for positive and ↓ for negative).

Apart from recommendations, the app provides to patient the level of adherence; awards; feedback; and alerts, as well as specific information about the CPAP performance. Finally, through a Web application, lung specialists may access to the system and take a look to the state of a given patient.

4   Conclusions and Future Work

IoT, as a set of existing and emerging technologies, notions and services, can provide many solutions to delivery of healthcare systems and services to empower patients providing better care and remote monitoring. In this context,

---

[2] http://www.resmed.com/us/en/consumer/products/devices/airsense-10-cpap.html.

we presented an IoT-based system aimed at remotely support patients suffering Obstructive Sleep Apnea.

Clinical trials just started. In the near future we will refine the system improving the intelligent monitoring system by relying with more data and getting direct feedback from patients involved in the experiments. According to an iterative co-design approach we will also work together with lung specialists to improve and extend the set of recommendations.

Acknowledgments. The study was partly funded by the Spanish Ministry of Economy and Competitiveness in the framework of the call "Collaboration Challenges" in the State Program for Research, Development and Innovation Oriented to Societal Challenges (Project myOSA, RTC-2014-3138-1) and the CONNECARE project (grant agreement no. 689802 - H2020-EU.3.1).

References

1. Atzori, L., Iera, A., Morabito, G.: The internet of things: a survey. Comput. Netw. **54**(15), 2787–2805 (2010)
2. Barrett, M.J., et al.: Patient Self-management Tools: An Overview. California Healthcare Foundation, Oakland (2005)
3. Kumar, K.C.: A new methodology for monitoring OSA patients based on IoT. Int. J. Innovative Res. Dev. **5**(2) (2016). ISSN 2278–0211
4. Resnick, P., Varian, H.R.: Recommender systems. Commun. ACM **40**(3), 56–58 (1997)
5. Strollo Jr., P.J., Rogers, R.M.: Obstructive sleep apnea. New Engl. J. Med. **334**(2), 99–104 (1996)
6. Vandenberghe, B., Geerts, D.: Sleep monitoring tools at home and in the hospital: bridging quantified self and clinical sleep research. In: 2015 9th International Conference on Pervasive Computing Technologies for Healthcare (PervasiveHealth), pp. 153–160. IEEE (2015)
7. Velickovski, F., Ceccaroni, L., Roca, J., Burgos, F., Galdiz, J.B., Nueria, M., Lluch-Ariet, M.: Clinical decision support systems (CDSS) for preventive management of COPD patients. BMC J. Transl. Med. **12**(S2), S9 (2014)

An Aggregation Plateform for IoT-Based Healthcare: Illustration for Bioimpedancemetry, Temperature and Fatigue Level Monitoring

Antoine Jamin[1], Jean-Baptiste Fasquel[1(✉)], Mehdi Lhommeau[1], Eva Cornet[2], Sophie Abadie-Lacourtoisie[4], Samir Henni[1,3], and Georges Leftheriotis[3]

[1] LARIS-ISTIA, Université d'Angers,
62 Avenue notre Dame du Lac, 49000 Angers, France
jean-baptiste.fasquel@univ-angers.fr
[2] Bioparhom, 89 rue Pierre et Marie Curie, 73290 La Motte Servolex, France
[3] Vascular Department and MITOVASC,
University Hospital Center of Angers, Angers, France
[4] Paul Papin Center, Institute of Cancer Research in Western France, Angers, France

Abstract. In this paper, we detail an in-home aggregation plateform for monitoring physiological parameters, and involving two objective physical sensors (bio-impedanceter and thermometer) and a subjective one (fatigue level perceived by the patient). This plateform uses modern IoT-related technologies such as embedded systems (Raspberry Pi and Arduino) and the MQTT communication protocol. Compared to many related works, monitoring is enterely achieved using a box as a central element, while the mobile device (tablet) is only used for controlling the acquisition procedure using a simple web browser, without any specific application. An example of a time stamped set of acquired data is shown, based on the in-home monitoring of healthy volunteers.

Keywords: IoT · Healthcare · Bio-impedancemetry · MQTT · Raspberry Pi · Arduino

1 Introduction

Internet of Things is a new paradigm offering a large number of possibilities, as underlined in a recent review [1]. In healthcare (see the recent overview [2]), such a paradigm facilitates the interconnection of medical devices and data, with various applications such as home tele-monitoring of patients or elderly people for instance. Many sensors are now available for monitoring many parameters (e.g. heart rate, blood flow, blood pressure, temperature, muscle contraction, weight...) with various technologies and distributed software architectures for communication purposes.

This paper focuses on the conception of an in-home aggregation plateform.

The main contribution regards the detailed description of both hardware and software aspects of the particular plateform that we developed, including various

© ICST Institute for Computer Sciences, Social Informatics and Telecommunications Engineering 2016
M.U. Ahmed et al. (Eds.): HealthyIoT 2016, LNICST 187, pp. 125–130, 2016.
DOI: 10.1007/978-3-319-51234-1_20

devices such as tablet, two particular sensors and the coupling of both Raspberry Pi and Arduino embedded systems. Our purpose is to show how such a plateform can be developed for specific applications. A part of this contribution regards the use of the MQTT protocol [3], particularly appropriated for IoT-based applications although rarely considered in healthcare, as recently underlined [4].

Another part of the contribution concerns the heterogeneous nature of monitored parameters: we consider both two objective parameters (i.e. measured by sensors) and a subjective one (fatigue level - can be considered as a subjective sensor). In our opinion, most IoT-based healthcare system focus on physical sensors although, for healthcare, additional subjective parameters such as fatigue level, pain level, ... may be meaningful from a clinical point of view. In this paper, note that we also consider a bioimpedancemeter, such a sensor being rarely considered (e.g. compared to previously mentioned sensors).

Section 2 briefly presents an overview of the developed system, while Sect. 3 focuses on its hardware and software architecture. Section 4 aims at discussing some aspects of this work.

2   System Overview

Figure 1 provides an overview of the proposed plateform, including a bioimpedancemeter, a temperature sensor, a mobile device (tablet) and a box for aggregating data and then posting them to the database using the MQTT communication protocol [3].

The bioimpedancemeter (Z-metrix developed by Bioparhom [5]) allows the measurement of various physiological parameters (fat mass, lean mass, total body water, extracellular water, ...).

The temperature sensor is part of the e-health sensor plateform developed by cooking-hacks [6]. Although the box is conceived to plug 10 sensors (i.e. ECG, SPO2, EMG, ...), only the temperature sensor is considered in the paper.

The mobile device is used to interacts with the box using a web browser. This allows to enter parameters that are required to perform measurements (weight and height in our case, being required for fat mass computation using bioimpedancemetry). The mobile device also enables to trigger measurements (i.e. bioimpedancemetry and temperature), acquired values being finally returned and rendered. Other information, useful for health state monitoring, can be entered by the patient, regardless any sensor (subjective sensor mentioned in the introduction). In our case, this concerns the fatigue level (value ranging from 0 to 100). Figure 1-bottom-left provides two snap-shots of the web browser, at the beginning (top) and at the end (bottom) of the acquisition procedure, with acquired values and a transmission acknowledgement.

All these components (temperature, bioimpedancemeter, mobile device) communicate through the central element: the "box". The box aggregates all data (measurements from sensors, information entered by the patient such as the fatigue level) and post them to a distant database (Fig. 1-B) using the MQTT communication protocol.

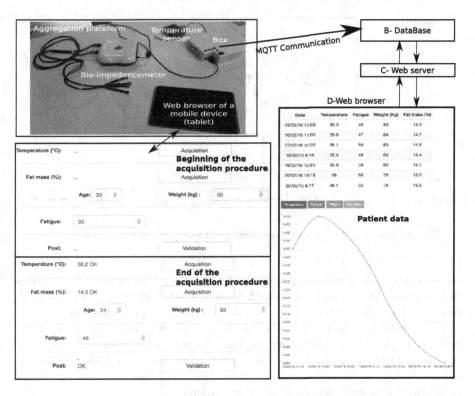

Fig. 1. Overview of the developed aggregation plateform (A) integrated a box (core element) and several external devices. This plateform communicates with a distant database (B) using the MQTT communication protocol, the content of which being rendered to render data within a web browser (D) thanks to web server (C).

A web server (Fig. 1-C) can finally be used to access to information stored in the database, for rendering purposes. Figure 1-D provides a snapshot of such rendering (time stamped measurements) thanks to the dedicated web server we developed.

3 Software and Hardware Architecture

Figure 2 provides a synthetic view of the implemented architecture. Section 3.1 details the composition of box, and Sect. 3.2 concerns the MQTT protocol.

3.1 Aggregation Plateform

In terms of hardware, the box mainly includes a Raspberry Pi and an Arduino controller together with the Arduino shield developed by Cooking Hacks,

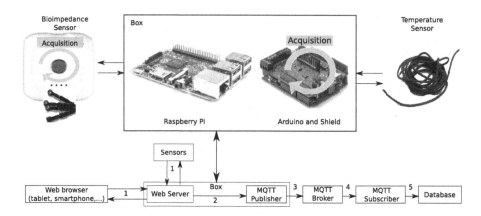

Fig. 2. Architecture overview, including software and hardware components.

for plugging related sensors (in particular the temperature sensor). The bio-impedancemeter is connected through a wired USB connection. Additional elements are packaged within the box (not detailed for clarity), such as two wifi dongles for communication (with the mobile device and with the database), a battery and an energy management system, so that the box can work in an autonomous manner. Note that, as underlined in Sect. 4, communication with sensors and mobile device can be modified or extended (e.g. both bio-impedancemeter and mobile device support bluetooth communication).

In terms of software, a web server runs on the Raspberry Pi so that the mobile device can get connected to the box using a web browser. Figure 2-1 models interactions between the mobile device (web browser) and the web server. It also models interactions between the web server and underlying sensors (i.e. acquisition is parameterized and triggered from the web browser as illustrated by Fig. 1-bottom-left). A REST architecture is considered for web server: each REST resource corresponds to a specific item (i.e. bioimpedancemetry, temperature, fatigue level), with related specific code, ensuring the separation of concerns and the modularity of the application. Note that the specific code related to the bioimpedancemetry embeds fat mass computation from electrical values returned by the sensor. For the temperature sensor, the related REST resource interacts with the Arduino board managing the acquisition (using the library developed by Cooking Hacks [6]).

When the acquisition procedure ends, the user triggers (dedicated REST resource) the post of the data to the distant database using MQTT.

All codes running on the Raspberry Pi are written with the Python language (web server, fat mass computation, communication with the Arduino and database with MQTT), using appropriate libraries.

3.2   MQTT

The principle and features of the MQTT protocol are described in [3] and has been recently considered in the context of healthcare [4]. Such a technology is particularly useful in the field of internet of things. One of the main feature is the related small code footprint and required network bandwidth.

Such a protocol is based on three elements: the publisher, the subscriber and the broker. The publisher publishes information on a certain topic, the subscriber subscribes to (a) topic(s) and receives related published messages. The intermediate entity is the broker, known by both subscribers and publishers. The broker filters all incoming messages and distributes them according to the topic and the subscriptions. Data exchange can be secured thanks to both encryption and authentication mechanisms, this being crucial for healthcare systems.

In our case, a topic corresponds to a patient (specific patient identifier). When the acquisition procedure ends, a REST resource triggers the diffusion (Fig. 2-2) of the acquired data on the related topic to the broker (Fig. 2-3). The subscriber receives the message (Fig. 2-4) and updates the database (Fig. 2-5).

4   Discussion

This system has been used by healthy volunteers for testing purposes. Acquisitions have been done daily for home during a couple of days. A single distant computer has been considered for running the broker (Mosquitto), the subscriber (Python), the database (MongoDB) and webserver (NodeJS): Fig. 1-bottom-right provides a snap-shot of the monitored data.

Hereafter, we shortly discuss two aspects: the use of a dedicated aggregator rather than the mobile device, and the ability to integrate additional sensors.

Many recent related works consider a mobile device instead of a dedicated aggregator [4, 7] (the mobile device plays the role of aggregator and communicates with the distant broker). For instance, in [4] the mobile device acquires data from ECG and Oxymeter sensors using Bluetooth and a dedicated Android application. The mobile device also embeds the code for publishing data using the MQTT protocol. The advantage of such architecture is that no dedicated box is required, only a dedicated Android application is needed. In our sense, the main drawback of such architecture concerns the communication with sensors: although most mobile devices provide many communication components (e.g. wifi, sim, bluetooth, nfc, ...), their main limitation concerns the limited number of wired connections. In our case, as the local server considered in [8], the use of a box offering more connectivity (in particular wired connection) is therefore a relevant alternative. This furthermore allows to decouple the personal mobile device of the patient (e.g. including a GSM connection for general purpose and personal use) from the device used for health monitoring (e.g. which could provide another GSM connection but dedicated to health monitoring). Despite connectivity, such an aggregator involves a dedicated system no only for receiving data but also for performing computations such as fat mass in our case (possible using personal mobile device but at the cost of additional energy consumption). Our proposal has similarities with the local server presented in [8].

In terms of evolutivity, any new sensor can be integrated within the proposed plateform by connected the device to the Raspberry Pi either a wired connection, or a wireless connection (e.g. bluetooth). At software level, this involves the integration of the corresponding REST resource to web server running on the Raspberry Pi (binding between the tablet and physical sensor). The mobile device basically remains a "touch screen" interacting with the box (through the web browser).

5 Conclusion

This work provides a detailed example of in-home aggregation plateform using standard modern technologies. Next steps will concern the exploitation of this system real healthcare applications.

Acknowledgement. This work is granted by the french league against cancer ("ligue contre le cancer 49"), with clinical trials identifier NCT02161978. Authors thank Franck Mercier, research engineer at LARIS-ISTIA-University of Angers, for the development of some hardware elements of the box. Thanks to the students of the engineering school ISTIA who participated to software developments: Mehdi Bellaj, Pierre Cochard, Mathieu Colas, Antoine Jouet, Audrey Lebret, Julien Monnier, Alexandre Ortiz, Dimitri Robin and Alexis Teixeira.

References

1. Borgia, E.: The internet of things vision: key features, applications and open issues. Comput. Commun. **54**, 1–31 (2014)
2. Yin, Y., Zeng, Y., Chen, X., Fan, Y.: The internet of things in healthcare: an overview. J. Ind. Inf. Integr. **1**, 3–13 (2016)
3. Message Queuing Telemetry Transport (MQTT). http://mqtt.org
4. Barata, D., Louzada, G., Carreiro, A., Damasceno, A.: System of acquisition, transmission, storage and visualization of pulse oximeter and ECG data using android and MQTT. Procedia Technol. **9**, 1265–1272 (2013)
5. Bioparhom. http://www.bioparhom.com/en
6. Hacks, C.: e-Health Sensor Plateform. http://www.cooking-hacks.com
7. Hussaina, A., Wenbia, R., da Silvab, A.L., Nadhera, M., Mudhisha, M.: Health and emergency-care platform for the elderly and disabled people in the Smart City. J. Syst. Softw. **110**, 253–263 (2015)
8. Mano, L.Y., Faical, B.S., Nakamura, L.H.V., Gomes, P.H., Libralon, G.L., Meneguete, R.I., Filho, G.P.R., Giancristofaro, G.T., Pessin, G., Krishnamachari, B., Ueyama, J.: Exploiting IoT technologies for enhancing Health Smart Homes through patient identification and emotion recognition. Comput. Commun., 1–13 (2016)

Posters (Short Papers)

Smartmirror: An Embedded Non-contact System for Health Monitoring at Home

Hamidur Rahman[✉], Shankar Iyer, Caroline Meusburger,
Kolja Dobrovoljski, Mihaela Stoycheva, Vukan Turkulov,
Shahina Begum, and Mobyen Uddin Ahmed

School of Innovation, Design and Engineering,
Mälardalen University, Västerås, Sweden
{hamidur.rahman,shankar.iyer,caroline.meusburger,
kolja.dobrovoljski,mihaela.stoycheva,vukan.turkulov,
shahina.begum,mobyen.ahmed}@mdh.se

Abstract. The 'Smart Mirror' project introduces non-contact based technological innovations at our homes where its usage can be as ubiquitous as 'looking at a mirror' while providing critical actionable insights thereby leading to improved care and outcomes. The key objectives is to detect key physiological markers like Heart Rate (HR), Respiration Rate (RR), Inter-beat-interval (IBI) and Blood Pressure (BP) and also drowsiness using the video input of the individual standing in front of the mirror and display the results in real-time. A satisfactory level of accuracy has been attained with respect to the reference sensors signal.

Keywords: Physiological parameters · Photo plethysmography · Heart rate · Respiration rate · Inter-beat-interval · Blood pressure and drowsiness

1 Introduction

Non-contact based physiological parameters extraction research was started almost 2 decades before e.g. in 1995 [1] and after a long gap the first successful experiment was initiated in 2011 by Poh et al. [2] which opens the window of non-contact based health monitoring system. Thisarticle focuses on design and development of a non-contact based camera system to detect, track and recognize a human face and provide individuals' current state of biological signals. The goal is to display the outcomein real-timeon a screen. As soon as the system recognizes a person it calculates the users HR, IBI and RR as well as BP and displays values on the output screen using a text massage. Also, the proposed system detects eyes and notifies the user about individual's drowsiness state. Additionally, the system can work as a personal reminder e.g., remind the identified person in a certain time of the dayto take his or her daily medicine. To set up the data in the database, the system has an independent web application for saving new reminders to a persistent database.

© ICST Institute for Computer Sciences, Social Informatics and Telecommunications Engineering 2016
M.U. Ahmed et al. (Eds.): HealthyIoT 2016, LNICST 187, pp. 133–137, 2016.
DOI: 10.1007/978-3-319-51234-1_21

2   Data Collection, Methods and Implementation

There were two different sessions for the data collection and in each session there were 10 test persons (3 Female and 7 male) of different height, weight and skin color. In the first session, facial video was recorded for all the test persons from approximately 1 m from the laptop webcam in normal sitting position on a chair without any movement in constant environmental illumination. Thephysiological parameters were extracted in offline and saved in an excel file. In the second session, physiological parameters were extracted in real time considering normal movement of the test person in varying amount of environmental illumination. In both the session a reference sensor systems called cStress[1] was used for the evaluation of proposed algorithms. The system was developed in Visual Studio 2015 and the programming language was C++. Additionally, we use several libraries that help us with implementation details: OpenCV is used for the image processing and for most of the detection, tracking and recognition algorithms. Boost is used for providing us with timestamp tool and threadsafe data structures such as circular buffers. Finally, ptheards library is used for parallel executions.

The system can be divided into three modules, namely input gathering module, face detection/tracking/recognition module and biological parameters extraction module which are operated independently in three distinct threads. The face detection/ tracking/recognition module works with the buffer that contains the raw frames and stores its result in several other buffers for cropped face, eyes and hands detected in the raw input. Finally, the module for biological extraction itself can be thought of like 3 sub-modules - one for extraction of heart beat, inter-beat interval and respiration rate, one for blood pressure and one for eye analysis. The first one works with the buffer containing faces and outputs to a buffer of foreheads, the second one - with the buffer containing detected eyes and the third one with the buffer containing foreheads and hands. In this way we achieve parallel execution and thus the frame rate is not reduced and is at its maximum capacity.

3   Parameters Extraction, Results and Evaluation

Three different physiological parameters such as HR, RR and IBI were extracted in the first phase in offline considering sitting position using the method used in [3]. In the second phase, again the parameters were extracted in real time considering normal movement and environmental illumination variation [4, 5]. A comparative result for these parameters for a test person is seen in Table 1. For BP, we calculate the pulse transit time (PTT) between forehead and the palm as Fig. 1(b) like [6].

PTT is calculated from the phase difference of the heartbeat frequency component of the forehead and palm video streams. However, instead of using a formula for calculating the blood pressure, we train a three-layer artificial neural network to determine whether the blood pressure is low, medium or high. In order to have the artificial neural network well trained, we created learning data set by measuring BP and

---

[1] http://stressmedicin.se/neuro-psykofysilogiska-matsystem/cstress-matsystem/.

Table 1. Comparative analysis of HR, RR and IBI

Sources	HR	RR	IBI	ΔHR	ΔRR	ΔIBI	%ΔHR	%ΔRR	%ΔIBI
cStress	69.4	18.8	867.5						
Only R	82.8	24.5	724.7	13.4	5.7	(142.8)	19.23	30.5	(16.5)
Only G	66.7	24.5	899.4	(2.7)	5.7	31.9	(3.93)	30.3	3.7
Only B	72.2	24.5	831.4	2.7	5.7	(36.1)	3.92	30.5	(4.2)
Mean RGB	69.4	24.5	864.8	(0.1)	5.7	(2.69)	(0.1)	30.3	0.3

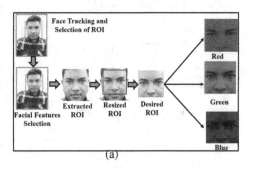
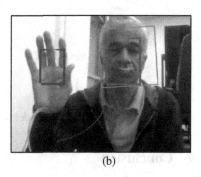

Fig. 1. (a) Overview of the image processing steps (b) ROI selection for BP

PTT of different people. We feed that data to an artificial neural network (ANN) which has four input perceptrons. The other three are obtained from the personal information database - height, weight and age. The ANN has three output perceptrons which correspond to BP being low, medium or high. We find the one that is triggered the most and select it as the final result for BP measurement.

For detecting drowsiness we extract six parameters such asPERcentage of eyelid CLOSure (PERCLOS), maximum closure duration (MCD), blink frequency (BF), average opening level of the eyes (AOL), opening velocity of the eyes (OV), and closing velocity (CV) of the eyes are extracted according to [7] and the steps are shown in Fig. 2.

These measures are combined using Fisher's linear discriminant functions using a stepwise method to reduce the correlations and extract an independent index. Here, fuzzy logic is appliedto determine drowsiness. From the facial cropped image, area of the both eyes are extracted, then each eye is separately processed in order to decrease false positive blinks and if person has ticks, it has been ignored. In preprocessing, RGB image of the eye is first converted to grayscale image, afterwards we apply histogram equalization on image, so binarization is easily done.

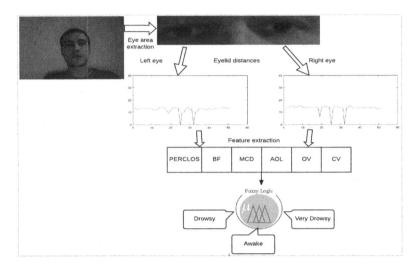

Fig. 2. Overview model for eye detection and drowsiness detection

4 Conclusion

The 'Smart Mirror' application developed to calculate physiological parameters and analyze the state of drowsiness was largely successful in performing the measurements in real time with relatively fast response times. The accuracy of the numbers obtained and verified by comparison with sensor readings was also satisfactory. Implementation of the improvements identified earlier in the paper would further improve the reliability of the system. The intent of the 'Smart Mirror' application being ubiquity, several improvements need to be incorporated in order that the system works under differing environmental conditions in everyday household and workplace scenarios. Possibilities exist to adapt the system for remote analysis and diagnostics, especially in locations where medical facilities are not available. Another applications area which may be explored is the determination of stress levels in the workplace. In conclusion, the 'Smart Mirror' application offers an intelligent lifestyle choice to society providing a means for improving the quality of one's life.

Acknowledgement. We would like to express our gratitude to all the participants, who give their time and data.

References

1. Costa, G.D.: Optical remote sensing of heartbeats. Opt. Commun. **117**, 395–398 (1995)
2. Ming-Zher, P., McDuff, D.J., Picard, R.W.: Advancements in noncontact, multiparameter physiological measurements using a webcam. IEEE Trans. Biomed. Eng. **58**, 7–11 (2011)

3. Rahman, H., Ahmed, M.U., Begum, S.: Non-contact physiological parameters extraction using camera. In: The 1st Workshop on Embedded Sensor Systems for Health through Internet of Things (ESS-H IoT), October 2015
4. Rahman, H., Ahmed, M.U., Begum, S.: Non-contact heart rate monitoring using lab color space. In: 13th International Conference on Wearable, Micro & Nano Technologies for Personalized Health (pHealth2016), Crete, Greece, 29–31 May 2016
5. Rahman, H., Begum, S., Ahmed, M.U., Funk, P.: Real time heart rate monitoring from facial RGB color video using webcam. In: 29th Annual Workshop of the Swedish Artificial Intelligence Society (SAIS) 2016, Malmö, Sweden (2016)
6. Parry, F., Dumont, G., Ries, C., Mott, C., Ansermino, M.: Continuous noninvasive blood pressure measurement by pulse transit time. In: 26th Annual International Conference of the IEEE Engineering in Medicine and Biology Society, IEMBS 2004, pp. 738–741 (2004)
7. Fathi, A.H., Mohammadi, F.A., Manzuri, M.T.: The eyelids distance detection in gray scale images. In: 2006 International Symposium on Communications and Information Technologies, pp. 937–940 (2006)

The E-Care@Home Infrastructure for IoT-Enabled Healthcare

Nicolas Tsiftes[1(✉)], Simon Duquennoy[1], Thiemo Voigt[1],
Mobyen Uddin Ahmed[2], Uwe Köckemann[3], and Amy Loutfi[3]

[1] SICS Swedish ICT, Kista, Sweden
nvt@sics.se
[2] Mälardalen University, Västerås, Sweden
[3] Örebro University, Örebro, Sweden

Abstract. The E-Care@Home Project aims at providing a comprehensive IoT-based healthcare system, including state-of-the-art communication protocols and high-level analysis of data from various types of sensors. With this poster, we present its novel technical infrastructure, consisting of low-power IPv6 networking, sensors for health monitoring, and resource-efficient software, that is used to gather data from elderly patients and their surrounding environment.

1 Introduction

In order to cope with our aging society, a current vision in the area of ICT-supported independent living of the elderly involves populating the smart home with connected electronic devices ("things", such as sensors and actuators) and linking them to the Internet. The mission of the E-care@home project is to create such an Internet-of-Things (IoT) infrastructure with the ambition to provide automated information gathering and processing on top of which e-services for the elderly residing in their homes can be built [2].

While the things need to communicate, wiring them is, however, unfeasible, inflexible and costly. Recently, low-power wireless communication has made tremendous progress. Today, we can network at least tens of stationary, battery-driven sensors and actuators wirelessly with a lifetime of several years using low-power IP-based communication stacks [6] on top of the IEEE 802.15.4 standard. In a smart home for elderly such communication means can be used to provide a reliable infrastructure consisting of stationary nodes. Stationary nodes are, however, not enough as monitoring the health condition of elderly people also requires on-body sensors such as physical activity and weight monitoring, blood pressure, blood glucose, heart rate, and oxygen saturation. Most of these sensors do not come with support for IEEE 802.15.4, but use Bluetooth—in particular Bluetooth Low Energy (BLE). This leads to a hybrid communication architecture where stationary nodes communicate with each other using communication protocols on top of the IEEE 802.15.4 standards while on-body sensors use BLE. For communication between on-body and stationary nodes, some stationary nodes are also equipped with BLE radios.

© ICST Institute for Computer Sciences, Social Informatics and Telecommunications Engineering 2016
M.U. Ahmed et al. (Eds.): HealthyIoT 2016, LNICST 187, pp. 138–140, 2016.
DOI: 10.1007/978-3-319-51234-1_22

Our healthcare application requires that in some situations, messages from sensor nodes must be delivered timely and with very high reliability. In the following we explain more about our architecture, which caters to these application requirements, and provide some initial evaluation results.

2 Architecture

The E-Care@Home software architecture, illustrated in Fig. 1, comprises different components that are built to execute in Contiki, an open-source operating system for the IoT [1]. To be able to meet specific application goals regarding metrics such as packet delivery rate, energy consumption, latency, and node lifetime, we employ TSCH (Time Slotted Channel Hopping MAC), one of the MAC protocols of the IEEE802.15.4-2015 standard [3]. At the routing layer, we use RPL [8], the routing protocol for low-power IPv6 networks standardized by the IETF ROLL working group.

Table 1 shows some results from our previous work [5], which reveals that even without centralized scheduling, TSCH achieves end-to-end delivery ratios of over 99.99 %. Hence, we improve reliability by two orders of magnitude compared to asynchronous low-power MAC protocols, while achieving a similar latency-energy balance. Furthermore, we can provide bounds on energy consumption. One of the challenges in our project is to extend the performance bounds to end-to-end latency and also include the on-body sensors that use BLE.

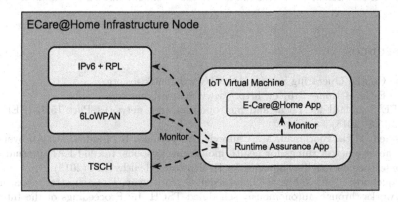

Fig. 1. The software architecture of static infrastructure nodes comprises a low-power IPv6 stack, built on top of TSCH. The application software runs in a virtualized environment that provides safe execution.

Another key component of the architecture is a virtual machine, which executes bytecode in a safe manner so that application software cannot exceed their assigned privileges. Inside the virtual machine, the sensing application executes and communicates sensor samples and system status to a base station using

Table 1. Performance of Contiki's 6TiSCH implementation on a 98-node testbed. RPL + TSCH data collection at a 1-minute packet interval [7].

	Delivery ratio	Latency	Radio duty cycle
Always-on	99.910%	126 ms	100.0%
6TiSCH Minimal (3-slot slotframe)	99.870%	349 ms	3.1%
6TiSCH with Orchestra Scheduler	99.996%	514 ms	1.6%

CoAP and UDP over IPv6. Depending on the type of sensor, the communication can occur at regular intervals or in response to events. Some health parameters, such as blood glucose and weight, are measured sparsely; whereas others, such as electrocardiography and respiratory rate, are measured continuously at specific time periods [4].

The base station, which collects all incoming messages from the infrastructure nodes and the on-body nodes, contains a sensor database, which stores all sensor samples in a structured manner, and which can be used to extract data for context-aware data processing and reasoning. Another application residing in the virtual machine is the runtime assurance application, which continuously monitors the main parts of the system, and ensures that the performance stays within the guaranteed bounds.

Acknowledgment. This work and the authors are supported by the distributed environment E-care@Home, which is funded by the Swedish Knowledge Foundation 2015-2019.

References

1. The Contiki Operating System. http://www.contiki-os.org/
2. The E-Care@Home Project. http://www.ecareathome.se/
3. IEEE Standard for Local and metropolitan area networks–Part 15.4. IEEE Std 802.15.4 (2015)
4. Ahmed, M.U., Björkman, M., Causevic, A., Fotouhi, H., Lindén, M.: An overview of the internet of things for health monitoring systems. In: 2nd EAI International Conference on IoT Technologies for HealthCare (HealthyIoT) (2015)
5. Duquennoy, S., Al Nahas, B., Landsiedel, O., Watteyne, T.: Orchestra: robust mesh networks through autonomously scheduled TSCH. In: Proceedings of the International Conference on Embedded Networked Sensor Systems (ACM SenSys), Seoul, South Korea (2015)
6. Hui, J., Culler, D.: IP is dead, long live IP for wireless sensor networks. In: Proceedings of the International Conference on Embedded Networked Sensor Systems (ACM SenSys), Raleigh, North Carolina, USA, November 2008
7. Watteyne, T., Handziski, V., Vilajosana, X., Duquennoy, S., Hahm, O., Baccelli, E., Wolisz, A.: Industrial wireless IP-based cyber physical systems. In: Proceedings of the IEEE, Special Issue on Cyber-Physical Systems (2016)
8. Winter, T., Thubert, P., (eds.) et al.: RFC 6550: RPL: IPv6 Routing Protocol for Low-Power and Lossy Networks, March 2012

CAMI - An Integrated Architecture Solution for Improving Quality of Life of the Elderly

A. Sorici[1], I.A. Awada[1], A. Kunnappilly[2(✉)], I. Mocanu[1], O. Cramariuc[3],
L. Malicki[4], C. Seceleanu[2], and A. Florea[1]

[1] University Politehnica of Bucharest, Bucharest, Romania
[2] Mälardalen University, Västerås, Sweden
ashalatha.kunnappilly@mdh.se
[3] IT Center for Science and Technology, Bucharest, Romania
[4] Knowledge Society Association, Warsaw, Poland

Abstract. The increasing ageing population worldwide imposes some new challenges to the society like the provision of dependable support while facing a shortage in the numbers of caregivers, increased health costs and the emergence of new diseases. As such there is a great demand for technologies that support the independent and safe living of the elderly and ensuring that they are not socially isolated. Ambient Assisted Living (AAL) technologies have thus emerged to support the elderly people in their daily activities, while removing the need of caregivers being always physically present in order to look after the elderly. The current AAL systems are intelligent enough to take critical decisions in emergency situations like a fall, fire or a cardiac arrest, hence the elderly can live safely and independently. In this abstract, we describe our solution that aims at integrating all relevant functionalities of an AAL system, based on feedback collected from representative users. This work is carried out in the European Union project called CAMI (Artificially intelligent ecosystem for self-management and sustainable quality of life in AAL).

1 Introduction

The independent and safe living of the ageing population worldwide is one of the major concerns of the present society [1]. Although there are individualized Ambient Assisted Living (AAL) solutions that provide fall detection and alarms, health-care monitoring and communication to caregivers, home monitoring, assisted robotics etc., there are few that can work as integrated solutions for AAL by delivering all the necessary functionalities, and none that relies on models that are analyzed for their quality-of-service attributes as well as correct functionality [2].

Based on the above, we formulate the following research questions: (Q1) How to integrate the various functionalities of the AAL system in a modular manner, to ensure flexibility and reuse, along with incorporating user preferences?, and (Q2) How to provide evidence for quality of service?

© ICST Institute for Computer Sciences, Social Informatics and Telecommunications Engineering 2016
M.U. Ahmed et al. (Eds.): HealthyIoT 2016, LNICST 187, pp. 141–144, 2016.
DOI: 10.1007/978-3-319-51234-1_23

To answer such questions, we have developed CAMI, a fully integrated architectural solution for Ambient Assisted Living, which incorporates the major functionalities of AAL systems, like health-data monitoring and sharing, supervised physical exercising, fall detection and fall alarms, smart home facilities, intelligent reminding and activity planning, and multi-modal user interfacing (graphic and vocal based UI), including the use of a robotic telepresence unit. The highlight of CAMI is its highly modular architecture, employing both local and cloud-based processing approaches. It follows a micro-service based approach, using message passing and inter-service communication in order to ensure flexibility. The CAMI solution will reconcile the increased demand for care in the current ageing society with limited resources, by supporting an efficient and sustainable care system. CAMI will be extensively tested and validated with end-users during our AAL 3-year EU project, which includes partners from 5 countries: Romania, Sweden, Denmark, Switzerland, and Poland [3].

2   Applications of CAMI

CAMI is an integrated solution supporting elderly adults with diabetes, cardiac diseases and mild cognitive impairments. The integrated CAMI functionalities are summarized below. (i) *Health care monitoring*: Health data are collected for preventive health measurements and monitoring vital signs; (ii) *Fall detection*: Fall detection sensors are used to detect falls and raise alarms; (iii) *Computer supervised physical exercises*: Advises the user to increase the level of physical activity; (iv) *Personalized, intelligent and dynamic program management*: Medication plans, daily, weekly and monthly program planning compliance and reminding; (v) *Report and communication to health professionals*: Health data communicated to both professional and informal caregivers; (vi) *Demand-oriented, personalized information and services*: Accessible through vocal and gesture-based interfaces.

3   Current Results

During the first year of the CAMI project, we have obtained the following results that address some of the issues mentioned in Sect. 1:

1. **Extensive user involvement:**
   - Primary (elderly), secondary (caregivers) and tertiary (third party organizations) users are involved throughout the project, from user requirements, through validation of concepts and functionality, to usability tests and field trials.
   - Shadowing and self-documentation methods have been used to acquire comprehensive data about the users, including body language, pace and timing in order to give a full picture of the world from the user's point of view. Differences and similarities in user requirements in Poland, Romania and Denmark are revealed by involving six users from each country. An important common aspect is the user's positive attitude towards accepting and using new technologies.

- A multinational survey with 105 primary and 58 secondary users has been performed in Denmark, Romania and Poland. The primary users group is composed of 49 males and 56 females respondents, i.e., 26 from Denmark, 42 from Romania and 37 from Poland. The secondary users group comprises 22 professional caregivers and 36 informal caregivers. The survey has identified both the requirements and the acceptance of the users for the CAMI components: (i) social interaction desired by 90% of the respondents, 67% accept Internet for this; (ii) 44% are interested in physical and cognitive games; (iii) 80% accept a mobile screen and 50–65% accept a robot.

2. **Modular architecture based on open source components and artificial intelligence:**
   We have designed a highly modular and configurable architecture based on micro services, which includes the following units: sensors, data collector, robotic telepresence, mobile phone, CAMI box containing a voice command manager, decision support systems, security and privacy modules etc., and cloud services. Points 1 and 2 address the research question Q1, of the Introduction.

3. **Current development:**
   The development of the CAMI components has started in parallel with the integration of: (i) Linkwatch, the intelligent platform for medical data collection and monitoring of patients in their homes (by CNet, Sweden), (ii) OpenTele, the open source Danish platform for health monitoring, (iii) Tiago, a service robot by Pal robotics, and Pepper the emotional robot by SoftBank, (iv) A multimodal gateway (by Eclexys, Switzerland), etc.

4   Future Work

Planned future work for CAMI includes the architectural modeling in an architecture description language, and the application of analysis and verification techniques such as simulation, model checking and statistical model checking to ensure functional correctness and critical QoS. These contributions target research question Q2. We will also continue with the development of micro services, implementation of interaction episodes, user testing and feedback. We also envision user premises field trials during the third year of the project.

Acknowledgements. Under the EU project AAL-2014-1-08, this work is supported by a grant of the Romanian National Authority for Scientific Research and Innovation, Danish Agency for Science, Technology and Innovation, Swedish Governmental Agency for Innovation System, Polish National Centre for Research and Development, and Swiss Federal Officer for Professional Education and Technology.

References

1. Rashidi, P., Mihailidis, A.: A survey on ambient-assisted living tools for older adults. IEEE J. Biomed. Health Inf. **17**(3), 579–590 (2013)
2. Kunnappilly, A., Seceleanu, C., Lindén, M.: Do we need an integrated framework for ambient assisted living? In: García, C.R., Caballero-Gil, P., Burmester, M., Quesada-Arencibia, A. (eds.) UCAmI/IWAAL/AmIHEALTH -2016. LNCS, vol. 10070, pp. 52–63. Springer, Heidelberg (2016). doi:10.1007/978-3-319-48799-1_7
3. Active and Assisted Living Programme, ICT for Ageing Well, CAMI project. http://www.aal-europe.eu/projects/cami/

Driver's State Monitoring: A Case Study on Big Data Analytics

Shaibal Barua$^{(\boxtimes)}$, Shahina Begum, and Mobyen Uddin Ahmed

School of Innovation, Design and Engineering,
Mälardalen University, 72123 Västerås, Sweden
{shaibal.barua,shahina.begum,mobyen.ahmed}@mdh.se

Abstract. Driver's distraction, inattention, sleepiness, stress, etc. are identified as causal factors of vehicle crashes and accidents. Today, we know that physiological signals are convenient and reliable measures of driver's impairments. Heterogeneous sensors are generating vast amount of signals, which need to be handled and analyzed in a big data scenario. Here, we propose a big data analytics approach for driver state monitoring using heterogeneous data that are coming from multiple sources, i.e., physiological signals along with vehicular data and contextual information. These data are processed and analyzed to aware impaired vehicle drivers.

1 Introduction

Automotive industries are devoting to develop autonomous vehicle, however, before achieving that final goal [1], we have to rely on human drivers. Hence, driver state monitoring in terms of distraction, cognitive load, sleepiness, stress, etc. is essential in the transportation research area. These states are identified as causal factors of critical situations that can lead to road accidents and vehicle crashes. These driver impairments need to be detected and predicted in order to reduce critical situations and road accidents.

In the past years, physiological signals along with vehicular data and contextual information have become conventional measures in driver impairment research. Physiological sensors signals, i.e., Electrooculogram (EOG), Electroencephalogram (EEG), Electromyography (EMG), Electrogastrogram (EGG), etc. become the part of big data biological process that are both structural and non-structural, and complex to analyze. Furthermore, vehicular data, e.g., steering wheel movement, lateral position, break, etc. and contextual data such as driving experience, time of driving, road condition, etc. are also vital measures of driver's impairments. Besides, in real-time scenario, it requires a trade-off among resources, for handling the stream of sensor data [2]. Moreover, the advancement of technologies such as Internet, cloud computing, sensors, and wireless networks consequential of generating huge amounts of data stream. Big data analytics is the process that extract useful geometric and statistical pattern, retrieve knowledge, and use for decision making by analyzing and understanding the features of the massive dataset [3, 4]. The challenges in the big data analytics are to manage, process and transform the extracted structured data [5]. Therefore, we propose a multilayer approach for physiological big data analytics that can be used for vehicle

© ICST Institute for Computer Sciences, Social Informatics and Telecommunications Engineering 2016
M.U. Ahmed et al. (Eds.): HealthyIoT 2016, LNICST 187, pp. 145–147, 2016.
DOI: 10.1007/978-3-319-51234-1_24

driver monitoring; where usage of machine learning and reasoning with artificial intelligence can facilitate the challenging tasks of big data analytics [6].

2 Approaches and Methods

A schematic diagram of big data analytics for drivers' state monitoring, is shown in Fig. 1. The first layer is the outlier detection and data cleaning layer. Sensor signals can often be contaminated with noises and need to be cleaned before analyzing. For example, EEG signals have gained increasing interest in mobile environments [7] such as vehicle driving, however often contaminated by ocular and muscle artifacts. We have developed a fully automated EEG artifacts handling algorithm called ARTE (Automated aRTifacts handling in mobile EEG) [8]. ECG can be cleaned using existing methods [9]. The next layer processes and creates structural data from the cleaned signals. Vehicular and physiological signals are time synchronized and resampled; categorical and quantitative information are retrieved and formatted from contextual information. Later, features are extracted from all kinds of data and signals, and stored for the data analytics.

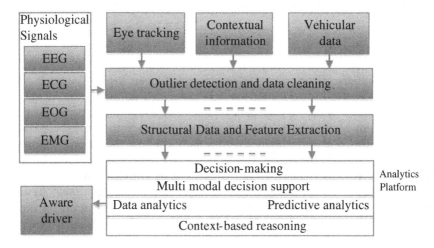

Fig. 1. Schematic diagram of proposed system

The core module of this approach is the analytics platform. The analytics platform is the combination of several sub-modules, i.e., decision-making, multimodal decision support, data analytics, predictive analytics, and context-based reasoning. Decision-making and data analytics can be achieved using statistical analysis, machine-learning algorithms. Data mining and machine learning tools and methods can retrieve hidden patterns in the data and also can be used for knowledge discovery [10, 11]. Deep learning based approach will provide classification and prediction from the data. Case-based decision-making is one possible use for the decision-making where previous decision come useful and will be integrated with the multimodal decision support module.

3 Discussion

Impaired driving due to driver's mental states, i.e., sleepiness, inattention, cognitive load, stress, etc. are one of the main researches of Safety driving in the transportation authorities and automotive industries. Most of the studies of driver's state monitoring are based on a single parameter, e.g., heart rate variability, eye tracking, or EEG signal analysis. Moreover, now a day because of the sensors availability, cloud computing, and IoT, datasets become huge in volume and also consist of a large variety in characteristics, and data are gathered with high velocity. In our study, we have considered multimodal approach, where several physiological signals, along with contextual information and vehicular data can be used to classify driver's state in real time. Using adaptable artificial intelligence and machine learning algorithms, knowledge representation, reasoning, and information retrieval can be handier and precise. Here, several sub-modules are combined within the analytics platform, using various machine learning algorithms that can provide constructive awareness to the impaired drivers.

References

1. Greenblatt, J.B., Shaheen, S.: Automated vehicles, on-demand mobility, and environmental impacts. Curr. Sustain./Renew. Energy Rep. **2**, 74–81 (2015)
2. Baccarelli, E., Cordeschi, N., Mei, A., Panella, M., Shojafar, M., Stefa, J.: Energy-efficient dynamic traffic offloading and reconfiguration of networked data centers for big data stream mobile computing: review, challenges, and a case study. IEEE Netw. **30**, 54–61 (2016)
3. Suthaharan, S.: Big data classification: problems and challenges in network intrusion prediction with machine learning. SIGMETRICS Perform. Eval. Rev. **41**, 70–73 (2014)
4. Leary, D.E.O.: Artificial Intelligence and Big Data. IEEE Intell. Syst. **28**, 96–99 (2013)
5. Cuzzocrea, A., Song, I.-Y., Davis, K.C.: Analytics over large-scale multidimensional data: the big data revolution! In: Proceedings of the ACM 14th International Workshop on Data Warehousing and OLAP, pp. 101–104. ACM, Glasgow (2011)
6. Maltby, D.: Big data analytics. In: 74th Annual Meeting of the Association for Information Science and Technology (ASIST), pp. 1–6 (Year)
7. Lin, C.T., Ko, L.W., Chiou, J.C., Duann, J.R., Huang, R.S., Liang, S.F., Chiu, T.W., Jung, T.P.: Noninvasive neural prostheses using mobile and wireless EEG. Proc. IEEE **96**, 1167–1183 (2008)
8. Barua, S., Begum, S., Ahmed, M.U.: Intelligent automated EEG artifacts handling using wavelet transform, independent component analysis and hierarchal clustering. In: Workshop on Embedded Sensor Systems for Health through Internet of Things (ESS-H IoT) at 2nd EAI International Conference on IoT Technologies for HealthCare (2015)
9. Kaufmann, T., Sütterlin, S., Schulz, S.M., Vögele, C.: ARTiiFACT: a tool for heart rate artifact processing and heart rate variability analysis. Behav. Res. Methods **43**, 1161–1170 (2011)
10. Condie, T., Mineiro, P., Polyzotis, N., Weimer, M.: Machine learning for big data. In: Proceedings of the 2013 ACM SIGMOD International Conference on Management of Data, pp. 939–942. ACM, New York (2013)
11. Depeige, A., Doyencourt, D.: Actionable Knowledge As A Service (AKAAS): leveraging big data analytics in cloud computing environments. J. Big Data **2**, 1–16 (2015)

Falling Angel – A Wrist Worn Fall Detection System Using K-NN Algorithm

Hamidur Rahman[1(✉)], Johan Sandberg[1], Lennart Eriksson[1],
Mohammad Heidari[1], Jan Arwald[2], Peter Eriksson[2], Shahina Begum[1],
Maria Lindén[1], and Mobyen Uddin Ahmed[1]

[1] School of Innovation, Design and Engineering, Mälardalen University,
Västerås, Sweden
{hamidur.rahman,johan.sandberg,lennart.eriksson,
mohammad.heidari,shahina.begum,maria.linden,
mobyen.ahmed}@mdh.se
[2] Exformation AB, Lidingö, Sweden
{jan.arwald,peter.eriksson}@exformation.com

Abstract. A wrist worn fall detection system has been developed where the accelerometer data from an angel sensor is analyzed by a two-layered algorithm in an android phone. Here, the first layer uses a threshold to find potential falls and if the thresholds are met, then in the second layer a machine learning i.e., k-Nearest Neighbor (k-NN) algorithm analyses the data to differentiate it from Activities of Daily Living (ADL) in order to filter out false positives. The final result of this project using the k-NN algorithm provides a classification sensitivity of 96.4%. Here, the acquired sensitivity is 88.1% for the fall detection and the specificity for ADL is 98.1%.

Keywords: Fall detection · Angel device · k-Nearest Neighbor

1 Introduction

Today fall-related injuries are increasing due to the increasing life expectancy. So, falls amongst elderly is a major global problem which has an expensive effect in the society. In a Swedish report from 2013 it has been shown that more than 270,000 fall accidents happened where patients had to visit the emergency room [1]. Since the risk of fatality increases by 12% if a person is not found within the first hour after a fall has occurred, fall detection system that both are accurate and comfortable to wear are urgently needed [2]. There are several approaches for detecting falls such as Vision based, wearable devices and other ambient devices [3–5]. In this paper we present a wrist worn fall detection system using a built-in accelerometer in an Angel (M1)[1] sensor device. This system consist of a bracelet that has several sensors and communicates with a smart phone with the help of the Bluetooth Low Energy protocol (BLE). We also present an algorithm using thresholds to detect all potential falls and if a fall is detected on the

---

[1] www.angelsensor.com.

© ICST Institute for Computer Sciences, Social Informatics and Telecommunications Engineering 2016
M.U. Ahmed et al. (Eds.): HealthyIoT 2016, LNICST 187, pp. 148–151, 2016.
DOI: 10.1007/978-3-319-51234-1_25

wrist worn device the buffered data is analyzed using the k-Nearest Neighbor (k-NN) [6] algorithm on the connected phone to confirm a fall.

2   Data Collection, Data Analysis and Method

The data collection was taken place by 3 male subjects of different age, height and weight using Angel sensor. A mattress was placed on the floor and a bench of equal height was placed besides the mattress, the test subjects were told to fall 10 times for each defined event. All the data from the Angel sensor is saved in a Comma Separated Variable (CSV) file and the application at the same time gather accelerometer data from the phone. Initially the raw data is visualized using a MATLAB[2] function which shows that the data from both the phone and Angel sensor follows 3 main phases as shown in Fig. 1(a). The first phase is rather stable state and falling toward the ground (the G-force drops before the person hits the ground), in the second phase the person hits the ground (the G-force gets very high for a short time and then bounces up and down a few times) and in the third and final phase the person lays still on the ground (the G-force smooths out and gets close to the gravity on earth 9.807 m/s^2). Comparing falls against walking for instance, which is one of the more common ADL that will happen during a regular day and it is seen that the pattern is repetitive and the distances between the lowest point and the highest is further apart from each other.

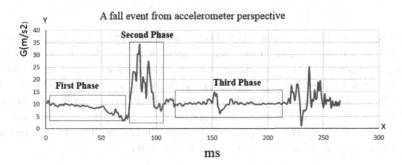

Fig. 1. Accelerometer perspective of a fall event

This knowledge helps when selecting and tuning the algorithms used later on. For the pattern recognition part of the fall detection system, the machine learning algorithm k-Nearest Neighbor (k-NN) was chosen due to its somewhat low computational power in comparison to other techniques such as neural networks etc. The strength of this is that the system can look at the similarities from other activities that it has been trained with and then make a classification based on the training data.

---

[2] "MATLAB Computer Vision Toolbox," R2013a ed: The MathWorks Inc., pp. Natick, Massachusetts, United States.

3   Result and Evaluation

The evaluation is performed by looking at the True Positives (TP) (a fall occurs and registered), True Negatives (TN) (an ADL is performed and a fall is not registered), False Positive (FP) (an ADL is performed but the phone registered it as a fall), and False Negative (FN) (a fall occurred but the phone did not register it as a fall). To evaluate the sensitivity, the total number of tests were 210, 10 falls per subject for every case and FN can be divided into two different types; one is Missed Falls (MF) which is when the threshold algorithm is not finding a fall and the other one is the real FN when the k-NN classified the fall incorrectly. To evaluate the specificity of the system, 8 test subjects were told to perform the different scenarios (ADL) as used in the data collection part. Each subject had to do the same activity five times which lead to a total of 160 cases. The result of the evaluation is shown in Table 1.

Table 1. The evaluation result

Features	Evaluation		
	Sensitivity with MF	Sensitivity k-NN	Specificity
No. of cases	160	141	160
TP/TN	141	136	157
FP/FN	19	5	3
Result (%)	88.1%	96.4%	98.1%

It is seen from Table 1 that k-NN algorithm is rather effective in differentiating falls from ADLs. This evaluation shows that the algorithms provide good result without creating false positives. The accelerometer based techniques shows that the system can work in a real environment. Devices worn on the waist are likely to add less interference by sudden movement when they are close to body's center of gravity. Since the angel sensor can be used like any ordinary watch it feels less intrusive and more comfortable to the user. However, it produces more sudden readings which need to be filtered out using machine learning i.e., K-NN algorithm.

4   Conclusion

Falling angel project aims at detecting fall in elderlies using Angel device with the help of machine learning on an android mobile phone. It pairs with a nearby Angel sensor via low energy Bluetooth and the results show a promising 96.4% correct classification during a fall event in the machine learning part and overall about 88.1% of sensitivity in fall detection. To our knowledge the application of a threshold algorithm together with a machine learning i.e., K-NN algorithm using a wrist worn accelerometer that work independently from the phone data is limited. However, the there are possible ways to improve the algorithm using experience based learning methods e.g., case-based reasoning.

Acknowledgement. We would like to express our gratitude to all the participants, who give their time and data.

References

1. Fallolyckor. Myndigheter för sammh ällskydd och beredskap, statistic och analys, MSB752. https://www.msb.se/RibData/Filer/pdf/27442.pdf
2. W. H. Organization: Who global report on falls prevention in older age. http://www.who.int/ageing/publications/Falls_prevention7March.pdf
3. Fahmi, P.N.A., Viet, V., Deok-Jai, C.: Semi-supervised fall detection algorithm using fall indicators in smartphone. In: 6th International Conference on Ubiquitous Information Management and Communication, ICUIMC 2012, pp. 122:1–122:9 (2012)
4. Fudickar, S., Karth, C., Mahr, P., Schnor, B.: Fall-detection simulator for accelerometers with in-hardware preprocessing. In: 5th International Conference on PErvasive Technologies Related to Assistive Environments, PETRA 2012, New York, NY, USA, pp. 41:1–41:7 (2012)
5. Vilarinho, T., Farshchian, B., Bajer, D.G., Dahl, O.H., Egge, I., Hegdal, S.S., et al.: A combined smartphone and smartwatch fall detection system. In: IEEE International Conference on Computer and Information Technology; Ubiquitous Computing and Communications; Dependable, Autonomic and Secure Computing; Pervasive Intelligence and Computing (CIT/IUCC/DASC/PICOM), pp. 1443–1448, October 2015
6. Altman, N.S.: An introduction to kernel and nearest-neighbor nonparametric regression. Am. Stat. **46**, 175–185 (1992)

RFID Based Telemedicine System for Localizing Elderly with Chronic Diseases

M.W. Raad$^{(\boxtimes)}$ and Tarek Sheltami

Computer Engineering Department, King Fahd Universtiy of Petroleum
and Minerals, Dhahran 31261, Saudi Arabia
{raad,tarek}@kfupm.edu.sa

Abstract. By 2020, it is predicted that chronic diseases to be account for almost three quarters of all deaths. This aging problem contributes greatly to chronic diseases like Alzheimer's. The major implications of Alzheimer are patient safety and care. The aim of this paper is to develop a Telemedicine system, based on Internet of Things (IoT) technology, for monitoring elderly individuals suffering from Alzheimer's. We describe a working prototype that is able to capture vital signs and deliver the desired data remotely for elderly staying at home, using wearable ECG wireless sensor. In addition, an Active wearable Radio Frequency Identification (RFID) wristband, with IR room locators are used to monitor the whereabouts of the elderly at room level along with an Android APP tool. This prototype was successfully tested on a number of patients at King Fahd University of Petroleum and Minerals (KFUPM) Medical Centre in Saudi Arabia.

Keywords: Telemedicine · RTLS · Electrocardiogram · IoT · RFID

1 Introduction

Demographic trends indicate rapidly aging population throughout the world, particularly in Europe. In many societies the proportion of elderly population (aged 60 years or over) is expected to double by 2050 [1]. The rise in aging population means a rise of people with dementia [2]. Telemedicine has the advantage of delivering high quality remote health care, thus avoiding unnecessary hospitalizations and ensuring prompt delivery of healthcare [3, 4]. The application of wireless telemedicine can be facilitated by the utilization of the mobile technology such as RFID [5]. Many systems for localizing Alzheimer elderly exist at the moment, such as the assisted GPS, which uses a combined GPS receiver with cellular technology. However, these systems fail to work in areas with no cellular coverage, such as rural areas. Other researchers use Indoor positioning using Ekahau Wi-Fi RFID active system. Nevertheless, Ekahau is complex and needs a complicated system of access points to locate the Elderly [2]. This paper presents a low cost telemedicine solution for locating Elderly suffering from Alzheimer at home using active RFID and an Android APP tool without the need of complicated and highly computational triangulation algorithms.

© ICST Institute for Computer Sciences, Social Informatics and Telecommunications Engineering 2016
M.U. Ahmed et al (Eds.): HealthyIoT 2016, LNICST 187, pp. 152–154, 2016.
DOI: 10.1007/978-3-319-51234-1_26

2   The Proposed System Architecture

This system architecture aims to provide a telemedicine solution for an elderly suffering from Alzheimer and staying at home. The elderly may be handicapped. Also relatives, who might be spread all over the world, would like to be in peace of mind that their loved ones are taking care of. We integrate a wireless ECG sensor with the proposed telemedicine system. A number of samples of ECG data are captured from a number of Elderly professors volunteers. Any deviation of the data taken from its normal range indicates the onset of arrhythmia and hence requires immediate intervention by medical experts [6]. In addition, the proposed system has an added value of Real Time Location System (RTLS) utilizing RFID technology on zone based. It consists of an IR-enabled 433 MHz, an active wearable wrist tags, room locators and readers that enable tracking of elderly patients suffering from Alzheimer at the accuracy of room level at their own home or retirement home. We assume that the Elderly home consists of three rooms for simplicity where each room represents a zone. An IR signal containing a user assigned location code is transmitted by each room locators. Room locaters are put to cover specific areas, like rooms, entire floors or closets. When transmitting RF location payload to a reader, the IR-enabled tags reports specific location data. When the Elderly moves between rooms, its tag transmits the new location that was received from the previous room locater.

IR-enabled wearable active tags get ID location data and then synchronize with room locaters. The active tag range can reach up to 35 feet and suffers far less interference than passive technology, Fig. 1. An Android APP is developed using JAVA to help the elderly beloved ones locate him while moving between rooms at home. A TCP link is established between the reader and the mobile for this purpose. Once the application is launched it will open a TCP socket and start communication with the reader. Once the reader scans the tags in its vicinity, the tag ID is associated with a specific zone where the Elderly is located in by calling a Google map into the APP to draw three zone circles or the three rooms, Fig. 2. The markers represent the scenario when more than one Elderly is living at home. If the marker is outside the circle, this triggers an alarm that the Elderly is wandering outside the safe zone. A successful test bed was performed in the RFID lab for localization.

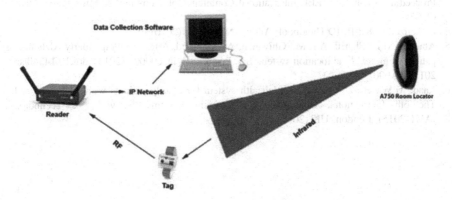

Fig. 1. Overall RTLS system architecture

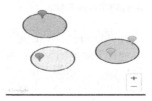

Fig. 2. Android APP for localizing elderly

3 Conclusions

The successful implementation and utilization of a wireless ECG system in KFUPM clinic has paved the way for establishing a ubiquitous mobile telemedicine system. The use of telemedicine provides high-quality service and increased efficiency to the practice of medicine. The use of active RFID & RTLS reduces the caregiver's burdens in a closed monitored home environment, helps them to monitor the movement of elderly suffering from chronic diseases and guarantees the elderly safety. Currently the wearable ECG sensor and wearable RFID wristband are separate. Ongoing research is under process to integrate them in the future.

Acknowledgement. The authors would like to acknowledge the support of KFUPM for this work.

References

1. Bujnowska-Fedak, M.M., Grata Borkowska, U.: Use of telemedicine based care for the aging & elderly: promises & pitfalls. Smart Homecare Technol. Telehealth **3**, 91–105 (2015)
2. Soon, S.W., Wei, L.T., Singh, M.M., Husin, M.H.: Indoor-outdoor elderly caring system. In: International Symposium on Technology Management and Engineering Technologies, Malaysia, 25–27 August 2015
3. Chowdhury, B., Khosla, R.: RFID-based hospital real-time elderly management system. In: Proceedings of the 6th IEEE International Conference on Computer & Information Science (2007)
4. Finkenzeller, K.: RFID Handbook. Wiley, New York (2010)
5. Abuhan, M.F., Shariff, A.R.M., Ghiyamat, A., Mahmud, A.R.: Tracking elderly Alzheimer's patient using real time location system. Sci. Postprint **1**(1), e00005 (2013). doi:10.14340/spp. 2013.11A0002
6. Raad, M.W., et al.: Ubiquitous telehealth system for elderly patients with Alzheimer's. In: The 6th International Conference on Ambient Systems, Networks & Technology, (ANT-2015), London, UK (2015)

Design and Implementation
of Smartphone-Based Tear Volume
Measurement System

Yoshiro Okazaki[1]([⊠]), Tatsuki Takenaga[1], Taku Miyake[1],
Mamoru Iwabuchi[1], Toshiyuki Okubo[2], and Norihiko Yokoi[3]

[1] RCAST, The University of Tokyo, Tokyo, Japan
okazaki@bfp.rcast.u-tokyo.ac.jp
[2] Ophthalmology, Tachikawa Sogo Hospital, Tokyo, Japan
[3] Department of Ophthalmology, Kyoto Prefectural University of Medicine,
Kyoto, Japan

Abstract. Evaluation of tear volume is important for diagnosing dry eye disease. At the clinical site, dedicated devices such as Slit-lamp Microscopy or Meniscometer have been used to quantify tear volume by ophthalmologist. However, these devices have access only in medical office and therefore have limited availability for the public. Tear volume changes with environmental, physical or psychological situation. For that reason, measurement of tear volume regardless of location, time or circumstances can be beneficial not only for healthcare professionals but also for patients. If tear volume could be measured by using smartphone, it is expected that the smartphone could be utilized as an IoT sensor for the healthcare application. In this study, tear volume measurement system was designed and implemented on smartphone. Further application for smartphone as an IoT device will be discussed.

Keywords: Smartphone · Tear volume · Dry eye · IoT device

1 Introduction

Dry eye patients have been reported to be increasing due to excessive use of visual display terminals (VDT), such as smartphones and personal computers. Evaluation of tear volume is indispensable for diagnosing dry eye but precise measuring is difficult because of the tiny amount and transparency of tear. Tear volume is considered to be associated with environmental, physical or psychological situation such as humidity, VDT work or mental stress. In the clinical site, tear evaluation is performed by shirmer's test, which includes placing filter paper inside lower eyelid, or by tear breakup time (BUT) measurement, which requires fluorescence instillation [1]. However, these measurements are invasive and therefore it is difficult to perform evaluation without any stimulation to the eye during measurement. Non-invasive meniscometer has been developed for measuring tear meniscus radius (TMR) which reflects tear volume [2, 3]; however, this device has been used only in medical office and therefore has limited availability for the public. If eye condition could be self-checked and controlled easily

M.U. Ahmed et al (Eds.): HealthyIoT 2016, LNICST 187, pp. 155–158, 2016.
DOI: 10.1007/978-3-319-51234-1_27

outside medical office whenever eye dryness or eyestrain is sensed, it could lead to the prevention of dry eye. Smartphone-based tear volume measurement system could be utilized as an IoT sensor for the healthcare application. Feasibility study of measuring TMR using the smartphone has been conducted in our former work [4]. In this study, tear volume measurement system "Meniscope" was designed and implemented on smartphone, and whether the system functions as an IoT sensor was tested.

2 Development of Tear Volume Measurement System

Tear meniscus (TM) is a thin strip of tear fluid with concave outer surfaces at the upper and lower lid margins and contains approximately 75–90% of the overall tear volume. In meniscometer, parallel black and white lines are projected horizontally to the concave surface of lower TM and reflected image from TM is captured. Then, TMR r is calculated by concave mirror formula (1) using projected line width t and measured line width i from detected image as shown in Fig. 1 [2].

$$r = 2 \, W \, (i \, / \, t). \tag{1}$$

Here W, i, and t are working distance between camera and TM surface, measured line width vertically against TM, and projected line width to TM, respectively.

Following this principle, prototype of smartphone-based meniscometer "Meniscope" was developed, where iPhone 6s Plus's (Apple, Inc.) display played the role of projector and front camera the role of image detector. Macro lens was used to zoom in TM and its attachment was made using 3D printer. Magnified image of lower lid was taken adjacent to the left eye by turning smartphone's torso sideways so that the display is located on the left. White, yellow and black moving bands were displayed in the monitor and reflected image from TM surface was captured. Examinee was told to gaze at the red fixation point on the display during the measurement. This system has W of 35 mm, t of 18 mm, monitor brightness of maximum, and line velocity of 33 mm/sec, respectively. TMR was automatically calculated by image processing algorithm including use of Hough transformation [5] as shown in Fig. 2.

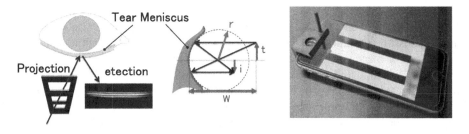

Fig. 1. Diagram of Meniscometry, edited image of [2] (left) and front view of prototype (right)

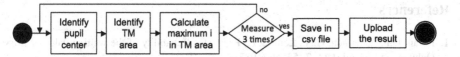

Fig. 2. Flow chart for TMR measurement algorithm.

3 Meniscope as an IoT Sensor

Preliminary study for 20 human subjects has been in progress for the purpose of confirming the feasibility of measuring TMR by using this system as an IoT sensor. A representative example of captured image during TMR calculation is shown in Fig. 3. We also have developed a system for uploading data to the server. It has become possible, with the prototype, to check the change in tear volume displayed graphically in the server, but to apply this system to IoT healthcare device, it would be necessary to combine tear volume with other data such as heart rhythm or physical activity.

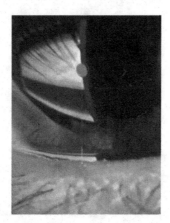

Fig. 3. A representative example of captured image during calculation of TMR.

4 Summary

Smartphone-based tear volume measurement system was developed as an IoT sensor by applying the principle of meniscometry. One limitation of this system is that it is difficult to adjust camera to the right position during self-measurement. In the preliminary study, it is expected that diurnal change of TMR will be measured using this system. The result of the study will be discussed in the conference.

References

1. Loran, D.F.C., French, C.N., Lam, S.Y., Papas, E.: Reliability of the wetting value of tears. Ophthalmic Physiol. Opt. **7**, 53–56 (1987)
2. Yokoi, N., Bron, A., Tiffany, J., Brown, N., Hsuan, J., Fowler, C.: Reflective meniscometry: a non-invasive method to measure tear meniscus curvature. Br. J. Ophthalmol. **83**, 92–97 (1999)
3. Bandlitz, S., Purslow, S., Murphy, P.J., Pult, H., Bron, A.: A new portable digital meniscometer. Optom. Vis. Sci. **91**, e1–e8 (2014)
4. Okazaki, Y., Takenaga, T., Miyake, T., Iwabuchi, M., Okubo, T.: Development of a practical method for tear volume assessment using smartphones. Trans. Hum. Interface Soc. **18**(3), 229–234 (2016). (in Japanese)
5. Yuen, H.K., Princen, J., Illingworth, J., Kittler, J.: Comparative study of Hough transform methods for circle finding. Image Vis. Comput. **8**, 71–77 (1990)

Towards an IoT Architecture for Persons with Disabilities and Applications

Jihene Haouel$^{(\boxtimes)}$, Hind Ghorbel, and Hichem Bargaoui

Higher School of Technology ESPRIT, Tunis, Tunisia
{jihene.haouel,hind.ghorbel,
hichem.bargaoui}@esprit.tn

Abstract. Internet of Things is revolutionizing human being daily life with the emerging of a huge number of connected devices. The potential benefits of connected things are limitless especially for persons with disabilities. Indeed, the number of disabled persons in the world today is considerable and their need of special care and adapted solution is a vital need. In this paper an IoT architecture for persons with disabilities is proposed and an IoT system dedicated to the visual impaired persons is implemented ensuring their assistance and security.

Keywords: Internet of things · Persons with disabilities · IoT architecture for PwD · Connected cane

1 Introduction

Internet connected devices offer a real potential to transform person's quality of life, particularly for persons with disabilities. This is also the subject of many researches and solutions. For instance, [1] propose a solution based on IoT architecture with mobile and M2M communication to help persons with disabilities to park. Also, [2] present an approach based on IoT in medical environments to achieve a global connectivity with the elderly and disable persons, sensors and everything around it to make their life easier and the clinical process more effective.

Persons with Disabilities have special needs and they require adapted solutions. So, dedicated solutions shall take in consideration their specific constraint such as mobility, safety of their connected devices. In this paper, an IoT architecture for persons with disabilities is proposed and a specific solution is implemented for the visually impaired persons.

2 IoT Persons with Disabilities Architecture and Components

As shown in Fig. 1, the proposed IoT architecture for persons with disabilities consists of six layers: Perception Layer, Networking Layer, Middleware Layer, Application Layer and two vertical layers: Management Layer and Security Layer.

In the Perception layer, devices are equipped with sensors such as temperature, humidity, etc. It collects data and send it to networking layer. The Networking Layer transfers the collected data from perception layer to the data processing system through

© ICST Institute for Computer Sciences, Social Informatics and Telecommunications Engineering 2016
M.U. Ahmed et al (Eds.): HealthyIoT 2016, LNICST 187, pp. 159–161, 2016.
DOI: 10.1007/978-3-319-51234-1_28

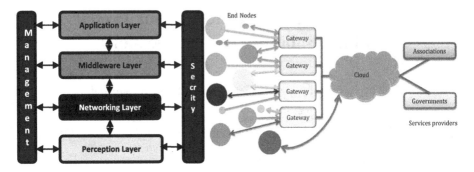

Fig. 1. IoT PwD architecture proposal and components

a specific medium. The medium can be wired or wireless. Middleware Layer provides facilities to applications to consume information received from the Networking layer. And finally the Application Layer, it implements a variety of IoT applications for many handicaps such as blindness or low vision, deaf, physical disabilities, etc. Management layer is responsible for the management of the four layers' components. The second vertical layer of the proposed architecture is the Security layer.

The components of the PwD IoT architecture, as shown in the Fig. 1, are End Nodes, Gateway, Cloud and services providers. End nodes are sensor nodes. We identified three types: active nodes, passive nodes and autonomous nodes. Gateway are devices that serve as link between the network of End nodes and the IP network. Because of the mobility of the disabled persons, the gateway can be a Smartphone or an embedded device in the PwD objects. The cloud contains a management platform of PwD and database server. Its main objectives are data storage and filtering, which will be used by web and mobile applications. And finally, services providers which are PwD Associations and government. The PwD Associations are suppliers of several web and mobile applications for the PwD and their family members. The government guarantees the efficient use of collected data to assist its different entities in planning of dedicated infrastructures such as roads, traffic lights, parking places, etc.

3   Implemented Use Case

The target handicap in this scenario is the blindness. The visually impaired persons face many challenges in navigating in many environments, which are often designed without taking them in consideration. In fact, the main used devices in Fig. 2 are connected cane, staircase beaconing device and connected traffic light. A web application is also implemented for visually impaired tracking by their family members. To receive alerts from the connected things (cane, staircase beaconing device and traffic light), the users are equipped with a Smartphone.

The connected cane in Fig. 2, is considered as an autonomous node in our introduced architecture. This cane provides several services to the visually impaired: obstacle detection, GPS tracking and water flanges detection. Obstacle detection is adaptable on two levels: up or down. Two different sounds are produced for each level.

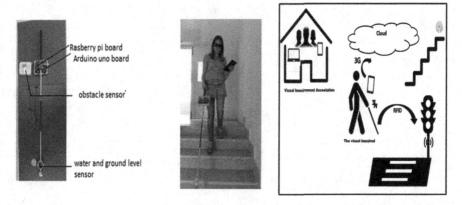

Fig. 2. Use case

The embedded board (RaspberryPi card) of the cane contains a GPS receiver. If the visually impaired person is lost, family members, who have the permission, will be able to find out his location through a mobile application. Finally, in case of cane loss, the owner can use an implemented Smartphone application to detect its location.

4 Conclusion

This paper proposes an IoT architecture for persons with disabilities and describes its different layers and components. In this work we also implemented a scenario for the visually impaired persons. Our work is still in progress as a lot of issues needs to be resolved related to the energy management and security.

References

1. Lambrinos, L., Dosis, A.: DisAssist: an internet of things and mobile communications platform for disabled parking space management. In: Global Communications Conference (GLOBECOM). IEEE, pp. 2810–2815, 9–13 December 2013
2. Valera, A.J.J., Zamora, M.A., Skarmeta, A.F.G.: An architecture based on internet of things to support mobility and security in medical environments. In: 2010 7th IEEE Conference on Consumer Communications and Networking Conference (CCNC), pp. 1–5, Las Vegas, NV (2010)

EHIoT Workshop (Full Papers)

Security and Privacy Issues in Health Monitoring Systems: eCare@Home Case Study

Thomas Wearing[1] and Nicola Dragoni[1,2(✉)]

[1] Technical University of Denmark (DTU), Kongens Lyngby, Denmark
ndra@dtu.dk
[2] Örebro University, Örebro, Sweden

Abstract. Automated systems for monitoring elderly people in their home are becoming more and more common. Indeed, an increasing number of home sensor networks for healthcare can be found in the recent literature, indicating a clear research direction in smart homes for healthcare. Although the huge amount of sensitive data these systems deal with and expose to the external world, security and privacy issues are surprisingly not taken into consideration. The aim of this paper is to raise some key security and privacy issues that home health monitor systems should face with. The analysis is based on a real world monitoring sensor network for healthcare built in the context of the eCare@Home project.

1 Introduction

With the development of new technologies such as mobile systems, embedded systems and wireless sensor networks, monitoring systems for healthcare are getting more and more common [1]. The rationale behind these systems is that elderly patients require systematic and continuous monitoring in order to promptly detect anomalous changes in their condition. Generally speaking, several wireless communication devices are employed and combined with medical sensors, to monitor elders from various points of view and according to different health parameters ([2–4] to mention only a few). However, the vast majority of the proposed systems are not taking into account what security threats the installation provides and which measures are needed in order to protect users' privacy. The security risks associated with such systems, indeed, can represent a high concern, because of the sensitive information these systems can deal with, like sleeping patterns, eating habits, heart rate and so on.

Methodology and Contribution of the Paper. In this paper we want to raise the awareness about the lack of concerns many solution providers show regarding such risks. To do so, we look at the main security and privacy weaknesses of a representative healthcare monitoring system, namely the home sensor network under development in the context of the eCare@Home project. The eCare@Home system is a made up of a collection of various sensors that monitor

---

Research partly supported by the eCare@Home project (www.ecareathome.se).

© ICST Institute for Computer Sciences, Social Informatics and Telecommunications Engineering 2016
M.U. Ahmed et al. (Eds.): HealthyIoT 2016, LNICST 187, pp. 165–170, 2016.
DOI: 10.1007/978-3-319-51234-1_29

movements and activities. The aim of this is to measure several attributes of the tenants and their environment in order to infer various properties concerning the health of the tenants. This analysis should then be provided in a user friendly format to care-givers. The motivation behind choosing eCare@Home as case study is that the architecture of the eCare@Home sensor network is generic enough to represent the vast majority of health monitoring systems proposed in literature. In particualar, in this paper we examine the possible ways in which an attacker could gain access to the eCare@Home system, what could be exploited and how the system could be changed to prevent such attacks. With this paper we also aim at providing some key advice to other developments of similar healthcare monitoring systems that will surely encounter the same security flaws.

Outline of the Paper. Section 2 briefly introduces the system under analysis, namely the eCare@Home sensor network. Sections 3, 4, 5 focus on the performed privacy and security analysis, identifying attacks and possible countermeasures. Finally, Sect. 6 concludes the paper.

2   System Overview

The eCare@Home health monitoring system has currently been developed in a fully-functional room configured to replicate a real world apartment, containing a bedroom, a kitchen and a living room. As sketched in Fig. 1, the system consists of several sensor nodes distributed in the apartment varying from light, pressure and RFID. These sensors are connected to a small board running Contiki[1] which then connect to a base station over an 802.15.4 network. Once the data has been transmitted to the base station, it is converted into ROS[2] format and passed onto the internal ROS network within the base station. Collected data is stored in the base station but in future revisions the aim is to upload such data to a cloud repository.

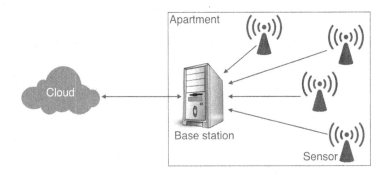

Fig. 1. eCare@Home sensor network

---

[1] An OS developed for the Internet-of-Things, http://www.contiki-os.org.
[2] Robot Operating System, http://www.ros.org.

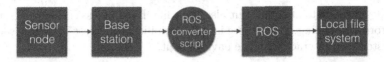

Fig. 2. Data flow diagram of patient data within the boundary of the apartment

To aid in highlighting areas of interest for the security assessment, Fig. 2 shows the data flow diagram concerned to the points of ingress and egress of the patient data. As mentioned earlier, the security assessment has been limited to the network within the apartment, as the method of uploading the data to the cloud has yet to be developed.

3   Wireless Communication

Attack: Wireless Sniffing. An observed vulnerability of the system is the ability to wirelessly sniff the communication on the 802.15.4 network. An attacker is able to use readily available equipment to promiscuously sniff the wireless network and gather patient data. This requires the attacker to be within a 10–30 m (dependent on device) of the location but it is plausible that an attacker could plant a device such as a repeater to extend the range or a receiver with significant storage. Both of these methods would allow the attacker to remotely collect the data without physically being within the 10 m radius. This type of attack could lead to a breach of patient privacy impacting the confidentiality of the data. It is noted that this type of attack would be highly targeted as it requires an amount of physical effort that would produce results on a small number of targets. With this assumption we can assume that attackers who are aiming to gather large amounts of data on a wide range of people will not see this as a viable attack. However due to the minimal amount of skill required to access the information it could be viable attacker for someone with a more personnel motive against the victim. It would be possible for an attacker to infer various states from the data that may be to their benefit. For instance, if someone is attempting to burgle the property, he can monitor the wireless network to determine if the occupant is at home or to determine the tenant's daily schedule in order to plan the best time for the malicious activity.

Attack: Spoofing of Data. In this attack, the attacker would require a more detailed knowledge of the system and protocols used but it is still plausible. It would be possible to inject packets into the network that are not genuine in an attempt to negatively impact on the patients data for the attackers benefit. This attack has greater implications when considering the future of healthcare monitoring systems, when such systems will not only have sensors that read from the environment but they will also incorporate actuators. These actuators may come in the form of embedded insulin pumps or pace makers. This means the security of the system does not just have to protect the confidentiality and integrity of the patient's data but also their life. Even in less severe case such as actuators for opening doors, there is still a significant increase in risk as soon as the system can interact with the environment.

Recommendations. As part of Contiki, the introduction of LLSEC provides link layer security across the 802.15.4 network [5]. This allows for the use of AES encryption across the network providing an added layer of security from sniffing. This method also allows for authentication and non-repudiation to protect from replay attacks. The authentication can be done in two ways, either authentication with a network-wide key or a pairwise key. The pairwise key is recommended as if that is discovered it will only affect the communication between one sensor and the base station where the network-wide key would result in all of the sensor data being compromised. This is a trade off between ease of deployment and security though, if the network-wide key is used it would be easier to enrol new devices as you would not need to setup a new key on the base station. For the encryption scheme AES 256 would be recommended but due to the low power environment this system operates in AES 128 would be a sufficient deterrent. Currently NIST still approve of using AES in CBC mode [6]. Key management for this network is somewhat difficult to balance, static keys within the network could prove troublesome as a sensor device could be stolen and have its key extracted from the flash if it is not made to be tamper proof. This tamper proofing though will inevitably increase the cost of each sensor. The use of certificates could help with this, each certificate would be unique to each device and could be revoked if the device is stolen. The trade off with this method is the increase cost of computing that is required as part of asymmetric encryption. Using certificates for authentication and then generating a static key between the two devices would provide a better level of security for the network. Unfortunately, this functionality is not currently available in Contiki's current build.

4   Base Station

Attack: Theft of Patient Data. In this attack, the attacker gains access to the base station by either remote or physical means and obtains the patients data. The current system stores all of its recorded patient data on the base station in clear text. This could result in the data being compromised if the base station is physically stolen or remotely hacked into. In the case of the base station being physically stolen the only data that would be obtained would be regarding that patient, so the return on investment for the attacker would be relatively low. However if there is a common vulnerability across the base stations then an exploit could be weaponized and used to easily access a large amount of patient data. This style of attack could be conducted by a rival company, criminal business or government agency as it would require a lot of resources.

Recommendations. It is strongly recommend to move towards and encrypted storage platform. For instance, data could be stored in an encrypted database such as SQLite this would allows for data to be easily written and read from the database whilst being stored in an encrypted manner. SQLite requires SQLite Encryption Extension (SEE) [7] to encrypt the entire database so that META data cannot be extracted. It is recommended to use AES 256 in OFB mode to provide the highest level of security using this framework. This does not address the base station being compromised but limits the impact of such a breach by restricting the attackers access to the information. Key management will be an essential part of the security of the system, deriving a strong key and storing it. It is not advised to store the key for the database on the base station but as these system will be possibly scattered over a large area it may be impractical to store the keys of site. Having a separate tamper proof key storage device connected to the base station can be a good option to get the best of both worlds but will incur an extra financial and maintenance cost.

5 Access Control

Attack: Unauthorized Access of Patient Data. In this scenario the attacker is an individual who has access to the system but is not authorized to access the patient data. Throughout the system there is an evident lack of access control, anyone with access to the base station can access all the data with no accountability. This is a detrimental to the privacy and confidentiality of the patients data. In the scenario where the application is deployed in the real world many people may have access to the base station such as carers, technicians and field engineers. Many of these people should not have direct access to the patient's data. To protect the privacy of the patient the access to the data needs to restricted so that only care providers and doctors have the rights to. Furthermore, this access should be monitored and logged so that accountability can provided if legitimate access has been abused. This type of exploitation would be far more likely to occur at the cloud level of the data storage. An individual who is allowed to access to patient data could steal a vast quantity of personnel data to sell to insurance companies or similar parties [8].

Recommendations. The SQLite framework supports access permissions so the DBMS could help control access to the raw data [9]. This will only be able to control access to the data that is stored on the base station but could be used to delegate different levels of access to different users. Logs should be forwarded to an external server as well as locally being stored so that tampering with them is discouraged. If the logs a merely contained on the base station there is the possibility that they will be modified or deleted. This access control and logging needs to be extended to protect the cloud storage as well. Indeed, the cloud needs a form of access control system that limits the amount of data the users of the system have access to. For example, a doctor should not be able to access all patients data just because he is a doctor, they should be limited to their own assigned patients. Logs should be stored and analyzed to spot any suspicious activity such as requesting large bulks of data.

6 Conclusion

In this paper, we have highlighted some of the basic security and privacy issues that a healthcare monitoring system should deal with in order to protect users and their sensitive data. The analysis has not been based on theoretical healthcare frameworks, but on a real-work healthcare monitoring sensor network developed under the context of the ecare@Home project. The main flaws we have identified are the lack of encryption on the wireless network used for the sensors, the improper storage of the patient data and the unrestricted access of the patient data. These flaws are common to the majority of similar systems proposed in the literature so far, as security and privacy are not sufficiently taken into consideration by the healthcare community.

Key recommendations resulting from the analysis includes: to secure the wireless network through available encryption schemes; for both storage and access, to use an encrypted database that can store the patients data in a secure format as well as control access to the raw data. This assessment is by no means complete as there might be still various flaws within the system. However, although these recommendations will not create a fully secure system, they will significantly improve the security of the healthcare system. Indeed, most of the attacks against healthcare systems performed in the recent years have been successful not because of sophisticated attack strategies, but because of a complete lack of basic security and privacy protection in the targeted systems. We hope this paper can be regarded as alarm bells for all the healthcare professionals, by sending out a clear signal regarding the need to pay greater attention to security and privacy of future home health monitoring systems.

References

1. Pantelopoulos, A., Bourbakis, N.G.: A survey on wearable sensor-based systems for health monitoring, prognosis. IEEE Trans. Syst. Man Cybern. Part C (Applications, Reviews) **40**(1), 1–12 (2010)
2. Tsukiyama, T.: In-home health monitoring system for solitary elderly. In: Proceedings of EUSPN/ICTH'15, Procedia Computer Science, vol. 63, 229–235 (2015)
3. Kotz, D., Avancha, S., Baxi, A.: A privacy framework for mobile health and homecare systems. In: Proceedings of SPIMACS'09. ACM (2009)
4. Dasios, A., Gavalas, D., Pantziou, G., Konstantopoulos, C.: Wireless sensor network deployment for remote elderly care monitoring. In: Proceedings of PETRA'15. ACM (2015)
5. Contiki Pull Request Containing A.E.S. Encryption, July 2016. https://github.com/contiki-os/contiki/pull/557
6. Dworkin, M.: NIST SP 800-38A, Recommendation for Block Cipher Modes of Operation: The CCM Mode for Authentication and Confidentiality 2002, July 2016. http://csrc.nist.gov/publications/nistpubs/800-38a/spp.800-38a.pdf
7. SQLite Encryption Extension: Documentation, July 2016. https://www.sqlite.org/see
8. Bloomberg: Your Medical Records Are for Sale, July 2016. http://www.bloomberg.com/news/articles/2013-08-08/your-medical-records-are-for-sale
9. SQLite, July 2016. https://www.sqlite.org/

Design of IoT Solution for Velostat Footprint Pressure Sensor System

Haris Muhedinovic and Dusanka Boskovic$^{(\boxtimes)}$

Faculty of Electrical Engineering, University of Sarajevo, Zmaja od Bosne bb,
71000 Sarajevo, Bosnia and Herzegovina
{hmuhedinov1,dboskovic}@etf.unsa.ba

Abstract. The paper describes design of a footprint pressure sensor system using 3M Velostat. The proposed design is intended for on-shoe implant for foot plantar pressure measurement. The system comprises Velostat based foot pressure sensors and IMUduino sensor node with Bluetooth communication towards mobile device running pressure monitoring application. The system prototype was implemented and used to test Velostat sensor performance. The proposed design has met all main requirements while providing fully functional and low cost solution.

Keywords: Velostat · Foot plantar pressure · In-shoe monitoring

1 Introduction

The objective of the paper is to describe a design of an IoT solution for in-shoe footprint pressure monitoring system using Velostat as a pressure sensor. Advantages of using shoe implants for pressure monitoring when compared to analysis performed using pressure platforms and walkways were recognized in the past [1]. There are developed systems using shoe implants that were customized for a specific research [2] or were based on commercially available implants [3]. Review of recent research in gait analysis shows that only 22.5% of research is performed using wearable sensors, stating that the portable systems based on body sensors are offering promising approach [4].

The structure of the paper is as follows: Sect. 2 describes application domain of the system and its requirements, with subsequent design of the system. The Sect. 3 presents Velostat and volume conductivity as a feature enabling its usage as a pressure sensor. Section 4 describes application for monitoring pressure changes and shows measurement results testing Velostat performance. Finally, obtained results are discussed and conclusions and recommendations for the future work are presented.

2 Footprint Pressure System

Feet provide the primary surface of interaction with the environment during locomotion. Thus, it is important to diagnose foot problems at an early stage for injury prevention, risk management and general wellbeing. One approach to measuring foot health, widely used in various applications, is examining foot plantar pressure characteristics. It is, therefore, important that accurate and reliable foot plantar pressure measurement systems are developed.

Pedobarography is the study of pressure distribution across the plantar surface, measured dynamically force fields acting between the foot and a supporting surface [5]. The differences in pressure across the plantar surface are the result of the distribution of the weight on the foot, showing the activity of muscles. In order to analyze the pressure distribution and foot biomechanics, the foot is divided in sub-segments, and frequently used sub-segment schematic is described in [6]. Sensor positions are defined to cover sub-segments of interest, depending on the application domain.

2.1   Application Domain

Typical applications for foot pressure analysis include injury prevention, improvement in balance control, diagnosing disease, sports performance analysis and also footwear design [6–10].

Improvement in balance is considered important both in sports and biomedical applications. Notable applications in sport are soccer balance training and forefoot loading during running [7]. With respect to healthcare, pressure distributions can be related to gait instability in the elderly and other balance impaired individuals, and foot plantar pressure information can be used for improving balance in the elderly [8]. Foot pressure monitoring can be used also for monitoring physical activities as weight loads while working [5].

2.2   Requirements for the System

Main requirements for foot wearable pressure monitoring sensor system are: light weight and small overall size of the sensor, limited cabling, flexible and light shoe implant, divided in areas for detection of pressure and distribution of weight. Another important requirement is also a low power supply.

Methods based on wearable sensors indicate importance of features such as precision, conformability, usability and transportability [4]. Majority of research in pedobarography is performed using non-wearable sensor solutions, what could be linked to cost of commercial implant pressure monitoring systems. This leads to conclusion that an additional important requirement is a low cost of the implemented system.

2.3   Footprint Pressure System Architecture

The architecture of the footprint pressure system is in compliance with common remote IoT health monitoring systems architecture. The proposed solution is a subset of the full architecture including: (1) sensor node: shoe implant made of Velostat and silicone with IMUduino device for acquisition and communication, and (2) co-ordination node: smart phone or other portable device with Bluetooth communication capability and application for monitoring foot pressure. The system is presented in Fig. 1. The proposed solution can be easily integrated with remote server unit for data storage and further processing.

Sensor node utilize IMUduino BTLE (r1.0.6) device with the following characteristics: Bluetooth low energy, Atmel MCU with 5 ADC channels, gyroscope and accelerometer, Arduino programming environment and small dimensions: 41.5 mm × 15.7 mm [11]. The IMUduino sensor node can be easily mounted on the shoe to acquire foot plantar pressure and movement data.

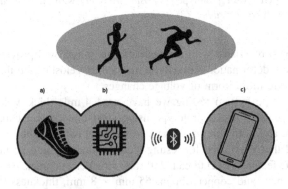

Fig. 1. Footprint pressure system: *shoe implant* with Velostat sensor (*a*); *IMUduino sensor node* (*b*); and *mobile phone* with application for pressure monitoring (*c*).

The IMUduino sensor node is equipped with the five AD channels enabling simultaneous measurement from five anatomic regions, as: heel, medial forefoot, central forefoot, lateral forefoot and toes.

3 3M Velostat

$3M^{TM}$ Velostat^{TM} is made of an opaque polyolefin, from the class of polymers, and it is impregnated with particles of carbon. Its chemical structure shows the current leading features, due to carbon particles. Physical properties are not dependent on age and humidity. Due to its polymer characteristics that change electrical resistance when a mechanical bending, elongation or pressure is applied, opens up the possibility of using this material in the pressure sensors.

The total resistance of piece of Velostat depends on its size, so it is possible, by changing the geometry, to modify a total resistance between two points. Increase or decrease in length, contributes to the increase or decrease of the total resistance, which directly connects the influence of pressure or stress on the measured resistance or voltage. Technical and electrical characteristics of the material depend on the thickness and the total area of which is used as a conductor, which provides the ability to create tape with different conductivity and thus sensitivity to mechanical changes.

For a successful detection and analysis of the distribution of pressure on the foot, when using a Velostat, it is necessary to make a segmentation of the feet, or divide the surface of Velostat in several regions, in order to have independent measurements.

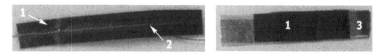

Fig. 2. Velostat based sensor prototypes: *Velostat track (1)* with *steel thread (2) (left)* and *Velostat track (1)* with *copper ribbon (3) (right)*.

Velostat should be coated with medical silicone, which will provide insulation to Velostat and allow deformation that will be mapped to Velostat, and therefore react to changes in pressure in the form of voltage changes.

For the prototype system testing we have used 4 mils thick Velostat (1 mils = 0.0254 mm). We have tested prototype using steel threads and copper ribbons as conductive pads, and both solutions provided identical results. The sensor prototypes shown in Fig. 2 that were used for testing Velostat linearity and accuracy, have following geometric features: steel thread: 250 mm with Velostat track 70 mm × 10 mm, thickness 0.127 mm, and copper ribbon: 65 mm × 8 mm, thickness 0.127 mm with Velostat track 40 mm x 10 mm, thickness 0.127 mm. Connection to the AD pins of the IMUduino device were made of steel threads length 200 mm, with negligible resistance.

4 Pressure Monitoring Application

Application for foot pressure monitoring is implemented for use on Android mobile device with objective for effortless data acquisition and measurement display. In addition to communication with IMUduino sensor node via Bluetooth channel, the application is responsible for communicating data for further usage via Internet.

The graphs in Fig. 3 present measurement results obtained during the system testing. The monitoring application is used to test linearity and accuracy of the 3M Velostat based sensors, and change in its performance depending on the wrapper material. The later tests were aimed to evaluate 3M Velostat performance when coated with different silicon types. The graphs are presented to illustrate different scenarios that were used during testing. The analyses included measurements using wrapper materials of different softness. The graphs in Fig. 3 correspond with the tests using softer wrapper material resulting in a less smooth pressure measurement curve. The tests indicated that change in measured value was proportional to change in the true value.

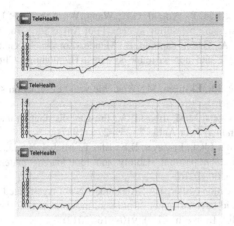

Fig. 3. Pressure monitoring graphs illustrating Velostat sensor testing: (*control mass - top*); *50% increase - middle*) and (*50% decrease - bottom*).

5 Conclusion

This paper presents design proposal for a foot pressure monitoring system using Velostat sensors. Implemented solution includes: 3M Velostat pressure sensor prototypes, IMUduino sensor node programmed to collect data from the 3M Velostat pressure sensors and from an inertial measurement unit with accelerometer and gyroscope, and mobile phone with Android application for pressure monitoring. The application is used to test linearity and accuracy of prototype sensors. Achieved results are demonstrating that the proposed solution is worth further development.

The proposed design has met the requirements related to the dimensions of the sensors and sensor node, while providing fully functional and low cost solution.

The solution is suitable for several other pressure monitoring health applications, and in addition to foot plantar pressure we are extending our interest in hand physiotherapy assessment and Kegel exercises. The later application requires only one measurement point. Different applications will influence sensor design and its wrapping. The future work demands custom development of the sensor node because the reduced number of measurement points enables more simple design and decreased dimensions.

References

1. Morris, S., Paradiso, J.: Shoe-integrated sensor system for wireless gait analysis and real-time feedback. In: Proceedings of IEEE 2nd Joint EMBS and BMES Conference, pp. 2468–2469 (2002)
2. Martinez-Nova, A.J.C., Cuevas-Garcia, J.C., Pascual-Huerta, J., Sanchez-Rodriguez, R.: BioFoot® in-shoe system: Normal values and assessment of the reliability and repeatability. The Foot **17**, 190–196 (2007)

3. Ramanathan, A.K., Kiran, P., Arnold, G.P., Wang, W., Abboud, R.J.: Repeatability of the Pedar-X1 in-shoe pressure measuring system. Foot Ankle Surg. **16**, 70–73 (2010)
4. Muro-de-la-Herran, A., Garcia-Zapirain, B., Mendez-Zorrilla, A.: Gait analysis methods: an overview of wearable and non-wearable systems. Highlighting Clin. Appl. Sens. **14**(2), 3362–3394 (2014)
5. Hellstrom, P., Folke, M., Ekström, M.: Wearable weight estimation system. Proc. Comput. Sci. **64**, 146–152 (2015)
6. Cavanagh, P.R., Rodgers, M.M., Iiboshi, A.: Pressure distribution under symptom-free feet during barefoot standing. Foot Ankle **7**, 262–276 (1987)
7. Petry, V.K.N., Paletta, J.R.J., El-Zayat, B.F., Efe, T., Michel, N.S.D., Skwara, A.: Influence of a training session on postural stability and foot loading patterns in soccer players. Orthop. Rev. **8**(1), 6360 (2016)
8. Hernandez, M.E., Ashton-Miller, J.A., Alexander, N.B.: Age-related changes in speed and accuracy during rapid targeted center of pressure movements near the posterior limit of the base of support. Clin. Biomech. **27**(9), 910–916 (2012)
9. Sinclair, M.F., Bosch, K., Rosenbaum, D., Böhm, S.: Pedobarographic analysis following Ponseti treatment for congenital clubfoot. Clin. Orthop. Relat. Res. **467**(5), 1223–1230 (2009)
10. Bennetts, C.J., Owings, T.M., Erdemir, A., Botek, G., Cavanagh, P.R.: Clustering and classification of regional peak plantar pressures of diabetic feet. J Biomech. **46**(1), 19–25 (2012)
11. Femto IMUduino BTLE Catalog. https://femto.io/collections/core/products/imuduino

Test-Retest and Intra-rater Reliability of Using Inertial Sensors and Its Integration with Microsoft Kinect™ to Measure Shoulder Range-of-Motion

Peter Beshara$^{(\boxtimes)}$, Judy Chen, Pierre Lagadec, and W.R. Walsh

Physiotherapy Department, Prince of Wales Clinical School, Prince of Wales Hospital, UNSW Australia, High Street, Randwick, Sydney 2031, Australia
{Peter.Beshara, Judy.Chen}@health.nsw.gov.au,
pierre@therealmsystem.com, w.walsh@unsw.edu.au

Abstract. This study determined the intra-rater and test-retest reliability of a novel motion-tracking system that integrates inertial sensors with Microsoft Kinect to measure peak shoulder range-of-motion (ROM) angles. Nine healthy individuals (6 female and 3 male, age: 36.6 ± 13.3) with no shoulder pathology participated following ethical approval. Participants performed active shoulder forward flexion and abduction to the end of available range. Repeat testing of the protocol was completed after 7 days by the same rater. Results demonstrated excellent intra-rater reliability (ICC = 0.84, 0.93) for shoulder flexion and modest-excellent intra-rater reliability (ICC = 0.82, 0.52) for shoulder abduction. A high level of correlation was observed between week 1 and 2 for flexion and abduction (R = 0.85 – 0.93), expect for left abduction (R = 0.60). In conclusion, an inertial system combined with the Kinect is a reliable tool to measure shoulder ROM and has the potential for future research and clinical application.

Keywords: Inertial sensors · Kinematics · Joint angle tracking · Wearable devices · Shoulder

1 Introduction

Shoulder range-of-motion (ROM) measurement in clinical settings is an integral component of physical examination to diagnose, evaluate treatment and quantify possible changes in people with shoulder pain [1]. Compared to any other joint in the body, the shoulder has no fixed axis and produces the greatest ROM in the body. Hence, the reliability of measuring shoulder motion presents a challenge to clinicians.

According to the American Academy of Orthopedic Surgeons, the reported average in adults is 158° for maximal forward elevation and 170° for maximal abduction [2]. Conventionally, shoulder ROM is measured using goniometry and the reliability varies, with intra-class coefficients (ICCs) ranging 0.26 to 0.95 [3–5]. Several other methods have been developed to measure shoulder ROM such as visual estimation [6, 7], still photography [8, 9] and smart-phone applications [10].

© ICST Institute for Computer Sciences, Social Informatics and Telecommunications Engineering 2016
M.U. Ahmed et al. (Eds.): HealthyIoT 2016, LNICST 187, pp. 177–184, 2016.
DOI: 10.1007/978-3-319-51234-1_31

Advances in miniature devices and technology have led researchers to utilise wearable inertial sensors to capture human movement. Inertial sensors consisting of accelerometers, gyroscopes and magnetometers have the capability to measure static and dynamic acceleration forces, angular velocity and the strength or direction of geomagnetic or magnetic fields. Inertial sensors have been validated for human joint angle estimation [11, 12] and measurements have shown promising results for various shoulder conditions [13–15]. Furthermore, inertial sensors have demonstrated excellent test-retest reliability (ICC = 0.76) and inter-rater reliability (ICC = 0.84) when measuring elbow flexion in stroke patients [16].

Microsoft Kinect™ (hereafter, simply 'Kinect') is a low cost, portable, motion-sensing device capable of tracking up to six bodies within its field of view. The device features a depth sensor which provides full-body 3D motion capture capabilities. Up to 25 joints positions are extracted in three dimensions for each tracked body. As a markerless system for clinical purposes, it is a favourable alternative to expensive optical systems inside the laboratory environment. To measure shoulder ROM in healthy patients, the Kinect has been compared to goniometry [17], photography [18] and other motion capture systems [19]. One feasibility study with 10 healthy controls reported the Kinect highly reliable (ICC 0.76 – 0.98) for measuring shoulder angles when compared to goniometry and a 3D magnetic tracker [20]. Similarly, excellent agreement between Kinect and goniometry was reported for active shoulder flexion (ICC = 0.86) and abduction (ICC = 0.93) in patients with adhesive capsulitis [21].

The Realm System (Sydney, Australia) combines 2 wireless inertial sensors worn on the wrists with an optical sensor (Kinect v2) to estimate human motion. Optical and inertial data are processed and merged in real-time to produce a full-body kinematic model of the subject. The integration minimises any weaknesses of both individual systems by enabling simpler initialisation procedures, a better visualisation of the estimated angles and better overall precision [22].

However, before such technology can be used routinely, reliability and validity needs to be reviewed to compare its performance to gold standard. Thus, the aim in this study was to determine the test-retest and intra-rater reliability of a system that integrates inertial sensors with Kinect v2 to measure human shoulder joint angles.

2 Methods

2.1 Participants

A convenience sample of nine asymptomatic adults with no history of shoulder pathology (6 female and 3 male, age: 36.6 ± 13.3) performed two shoulder movements according to standardised protocol, together with two raters (A and B). The same nine participants returned 7 days later to assess intra-rater reliability. The study was conducted at the outpatient physiotherapy department at Prince of Wales Hospital, Sydney, Australia. All participants gave their informed consent. The study was approved by the local Ethics Committee.

2.2 Raters

Rater A was a physical therapist of nine years, responsible for wrist sensor placement and initiating the protocol instructions. Rater B was responsible for setting up and executing the inertial motion tracking system with the Kinect. The same raters were used for both assessments.

2.3 Study Procedure

To measure shoulder motion, the system uses 2 WAX9 wireless inertial sensor units (Axivity, UK). The inertial measurement unit (IMU) is a small (23 mm × 32.5 mm × 7.6 mm) 9-axis sensor consisting of a 3-axis gyroscope, a 3-axis accelerometer and a 3-axis magnetometer with a Bluetooth Low Energy (BLE) protocol to wirelessly transfer inertial data. The sensors must initially be paired to the receiving computer, and the Bluetooth protocol allows for multiple sensor use. The pairing process allows for identifying and assigning each sensor to a specific part of the body.

Automatic calibration of the system established that the optical sensor (MS Kinect v2) was positioned at a height of 1.40 m and presented a tilt of −2.0°. Feet markers were placed at a distance of 2.50 m from the optical sensor to ensure consistency with the initial participant placement. Two IMU's mounted in a wrist band of silicone material were applied around the wrist using the ulnar styloid as a landmark. All participants performed two active motions: shoulder flexion and abduction in the standing position (Fig. 1). Instructions were verbally standardised and participants were asked to move their arm as far as they could. They repeated each motion 3 times at a comfortable speed.

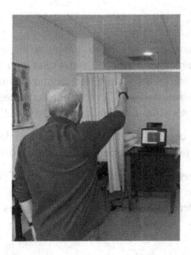
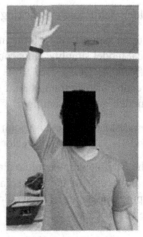

Fig. 1. Experimental setup. The measurement of forward flexion and abduction under instruction from rater.

2.4   Optical and Inertial Data Fusion

Orientation quaternions are calculated on the IMU sensors' microchip at an internal sampling rate of 200 Hz. Joint position data are extracted by the Kinect sensor at a sampling rate of 30 Hz. Both data sets are merged and fed into a full-body kinematic model describing a segmental representation of the skeleton using 16 limbs and 20 joints. The current implementation of the kinematic model ignores fingers and toes segments. The algorithm processing the kinematic model incorporates real-time predictive analysis which relies on the high sampling rate of the IMUs to compensate for the low sampling rate of the Kinect v2 sensor and generate missing positional data when the subject is moving, resulting in the kinematic model being updated at a rate of 100 Hz.

2.5   Calibration and Error Correction

As part of the merging process, optical data from the Kinect v2 sensor is used to further correct any potential drift in the IMU sensors, using forearms positions and a correction weighting of 0.1. This also allows for automatically setting the IMUs' magnetometer heading which cancels the need for initial calibration of the sensors. Optical calibration requires calculating the exact height and tilt angle of the Kinect v2 sensor in order to accurately convert the Kinect's joint position into the kinematic model's 3D reference. Sensor tilt and height can be manually measured and specified in the system configuration. Alternatively, the system allows for automatically calculating these by capturing 3 points on the floor plane and generating the transformation matrix between the detected floor reference system and the kinematic models.

2.6   Shoulder Joint Angle Tracking

The shoulder is part of one of the most complex joints group in the body. The biomechanical model simplifies this complex joint as a ball-and-socket joint with three degrees of freedom (DOF). Due to its markerless nature, the motion capture system extracts the centre of each joint as joint position. Two 3D vectors are extracted from the kinematic model: $\overrightarrow{U_{SE}}$ representing a vector from the shoulder joint center (below the acromion process) to the elbow joint center (between the medial and lateral epicondyles) and $\overrightarrow{U_{SR6}}$ representing a vector from the shoulder joint center to $R6$, defined as a point on the 6th rib along the midaxillary line of the trunk. The position of point $R6$ is derived via projection of the mid spine point of the kinematic model following the trunk and spine orientation. The shoulder angle ∂ is defined in real-time as the angle between the two vectors:

$$\partial = \cos^{-1}\left(\frac{\overrightarrow{U_{SE}} \cdot \overrightarrow{U_{SR6}}}{\|U_{SE}\|\|U_{SR6}\|} \right). \tag{1}$$

The shoulder flexion and extension angles are measured as the value of ∂ while the subject lifts and lowers his extended arm along the sagittal plane. The shoulder abduction and adduction angles are measured as the value of ∂ while the subject lifts and lowers his extended arm along the coronal plane. The neutral position (or zero value) is defined as the moving arm being placed along the lateral mid-line of the humerus in line with the lateral epicondyle.

The position tracking capability of the system has been compared against the gold standard MicroScribe digitizer device (Solution Technologies, Inc.), for the tracking of the wrist, elbow and shoulder joints. Several positions were simultaneously tracked using the system and MicroScribe. Discrepancies were measured by comparing the norm of the movement vectors between sets of static positions tracked by both systems. The average difference found between the system's position tracking and MicroScribe was 2.35 mm. With the MicroScribe device presenting a standard error of 0.23 mm, this strongly indicates that the system is able to accurately track positions in space. Dynamic positional tracking accuracy was established by comparing the system's output to the gold-standard multi-camera Vicon motion capture system (Vicon Motion Systems Ltd.), via a study focusing on dynamic movements. On average, linear regression results of $R = 0.97$ were found across all body joints showing strong correlations between the two systems.

2.7 Statistical Analysis

Data analysis was performed with SPSS version 22 for Windows statistical program. The intra-rater reliability of shoulder flexion and abduction was estimated by using the intraclass correlation coefficient (ICC) model (3,1). This was used as the investigation was an intrarater design with a single rater presenting the only rater of interest. An ICC of ≥ 0.75 was considered as excellent reliability, an ICC of $0.4 - 0.75$ was considered modest reliability, an ICC of <0.4 was considered as poor reliability [23]. Measurement error was expressed in the standard error of measurement (SEM) and minimal detectable change (MDC) was calculated to establish absolute reliability.

$$SEM = SD \times \sqrt{1 - ICC}. \tag{2}$$

$$MDC = SEM \times \sqrt{2} \times 1.96. \tag{3}$$

Test-retest reliability was determined from Pearson's correlation R and the coefficient of determination R^2.

3 Results

3.1 Intra-rater and Test-Retest Reliability

Intra-rater reliability is presented in Table 1. Excellent intra-rater reliability were observed for right flexion, left flexion and right abduction (ICC = $0.84 - 0.93$), but results were modest for left abduction (ICC = 0.52). Table 2 presents mean and standard deviations for week 1 and week 2, R as given by Pearson's product moment correlation and the coefficient of determination R^2. With the exception of left abduction, a relatively high correlation was seen between week 1 and week 2 values for left flexion (R = 0.85), right flexion (R = 0.93) and right abduction (R = 0.89).

Table 1. Intra-rater reliability of the realm system (n = 9)

Motion	$ICC_{3,1}$	95% CI	SEM	MDC
Left flexion	0.84	0.45 – 0.96	1.61	4.47
Right flexion	0.93	0.72 – 0.98	1.16	3.22
Left abduction	0.52	−0.17 – 0.87	2.16	5.99
Right abduction	0.85	0.47 – 0.96	2.45	6.80

Table 2. Mean and standard deviation at Week 1 and Week 2, Pearson's R and coefficient of determination R^2 for both flexion and abduction.

Motion	Week 1 Mean ± SD (°)	Week 2 Mean ± SD (°)	R	R^2
Left flexion	175.80 ± 4.03	176.55 ± 3.50	0.85	0.73
Right flexion	176.10 ± 4.39	174.42 ± 4.15	0.93	0.86
Left abduction	175.05 ± 3.12	174.46 ± 5.46	0.60	0.36
Right abduction	173.72 ± 6.33	174.91 ± 4.64	0.89	0.80

4   Discussion

This study demonstrates that an integrated system of optical and inertial sensors can be a reliable tool to measure ROM of shoulder flexion and abduction. All measurements demonstrated excellent intra-rater reliability expect for left abduction. This can most likely be explained by a general inconsistency in abduction measures observed by the raters. Flexion measures were relatively consistent between and within participants, while abduction was less consistent, predominantly when healthy participants didn't reach peak abduction before lowering their arms. Hence inconsistent measures may be due to an experimental limitation rather than equipment- related error. This study has its limitations as we had a small sample size and did not assess inter-rater reliability, therefore, restricting its applications in clinical settings between observers. Additionally, concurrent validity should be established by comparing measurements to other methods such as goniometry. As a preliminary step to assess the reliability of the Realm System, all participants were healthy, therefore future results need to be replicated in populations of interest, such as those with shoulder pain. This is currently being investigated by the authors of this paper in a clinical randomised control trial for patients awaiting shoulder surgery. In conclusion, the Realm System is reliable to measure shoulder joint angles. Advancements in hardware technology; the miniaturisation of sensors; user-friendly software with Bluetooth technology and simple body-worn sensors makes this method desirable for health clinicians.

References

1. Muir, S.W., Corea, C.L., Beaupre, L.: Evaluating change in clinical status: reliability and measures of agreement for the assessment of glenohumeral range of motion. North Am. J. Sports Phys. Ther. NAJSPT **5**, 98–110 (2010)
2. American Academy of Orthopaedic Surgeons. Joint motion: method of measuring and recording. AAOS, Chicago (1965)
3. Mullaney, M.J., McHugh, M.P., Johnson, C.P., Tyler, T.F.: Reliability of shoulder range of motion comparing a goniometer to a digital level. Physiother. Theory Pract. **26**(5), 327 (2010)
4. Riddle, D.L., Rothstein, J.M., Lamb, R.L.: Goniometric reliability in a clinical setting. Shoulder Measur. Phys. Ther. **67**(5), 668–673 (1987)
5. Hayes, K., Walton, J.R., Szomor, Z.R., Murrell, G.A.: Reliability of five methods for assessing shoulder range of motion. Austr. J. Physiother. **47**(4), 289–294 (2001)
6. Willams, J.G., Callaghan, M.: Comparison of visual estimation and goniometry in determination of shoulder angle. Physiotherapy **76**(10), 655–657 (1990)
7. Terwee, C.B., de Winter, A.F., Scholten, R.J., Jans, M.P., Deville, W., van Schaardenburg, D., Bouter, L.M.: Interobserver reproducibility of the visual estimation of range of motion of the shoulder. Arch. Phys. Med. Rehabil. **86**(7), 1356–1361 (2005)
8. Chen, J.F., Ginn, K.A., Herbert, R.D.: Passive mobilisation of shoulder region joints plus advice and exercise does not reduce pain and disability more than advice and exercise alone: a randomised trial. Austr. J. Physiother. **55**(1), 17–23 (2009)
9. Ginn, K.A., Herbert, R.D., Khouw, W., Lee, R.A.: Randomised controlled trial of a treatment of shoulder pain. Phys. Ther. **77**, 802–809 (1997)
10. Mitchell, K., Gutierrez, S.B., Sutton, S., Morton, S., Morgenthaler, A.: Reliability and validity of goniometric iPhone applications for the assessment of active shoulder external rotation. Physiother. Theory Pract. **30**(7), 521–525 (2014)
11. El-Gohary, M., McNames, J.: Human joint angle estimation with inertial sensors and validation with a robot arm. IEEE Trans. Biomed. Eng. **62**(7), 1759–1767 (2015)
12. Zhou, H., Stone, T., Huosheng, H., Harris, N.: Use of multiple wearable inertial sensors in upper limb motion tracking. Med. Eng. Phys. **30**(I), 123–133 (2008)
13. Coley, B., Jolles, B.M., Farron, A., Bourgeois, A., Nussbaumer, F., Pichonnaz, C., Aminian, K.: Outcome evaluation in shoulder surgery using 3D kinematics sensors. Gait Posture **27**, 368–375 (2007)
14. Luinge, H., Veltink, P., Baten, C.: Ambulatory measurement of arm orientation. J. Biomech. **40**, 78–85 (2007)
15. Teece, R., Lunden, J., Lloyd, A., Kaiser, A., Cieminski, C., Ludewig, P.: Three-dimensional acromioclavicular joint motions during elevation of the arm. J. Ortho. Sports Phys. Ther. **38** (4), 181–190 (2008)
16. Paulis, W.D., Horemans, H.L., Brouwer, B.S., Stam, H.J.: Excellent test-retest and inter-rater reliability for Tardieu Scale measurements with inertial sensors in elbow flexors of stroke patients. Gait Posture **33**(2), 185–189 (2011)
17. Hawi, N., Liodakis, E., Musolli, D., Suero, E.M., Stuebig, T., Claassen, L., Kleiner, C., Krettek, C., Ahlers, V., Citak, M.: Range of motion assessment of the shoulder and elbow joints using a motion sensing input device a pilot study. Technol. Health Care: Offic. J. Eur. Soc. Eng. Med. **22**(2), 289–295 (2014)
18. Matsen III, F.A., Lauder, A., Rector, K., Keeling, P., Cherones, A.L.: Measurement of active shoulder motion using the Kinect, a commercially available infrared position detection system. J. Shoulder Elbow Surg. **25**(2), 216–223 (2016)

19. Nixon, M.E., Howard, A.M, Yu-Ping, C.: Quantitative evaluation of the Microsoft Kinect for use in an upper extremity virtual rehabilitation environment. In: International Conference on Virtual Rehabilitation (ICVR), 26–29 August 2013
20. Huber, M.E., Seitz, A.L., Leeser, M., Sternad, D.: Validity and reliability of Kinect skeleton for measuring shoulder joint angles: a feasibility study. Physiotherapy 101(4), 389–393 (2015)
21. Lee, S.H., Yoon, C., Chung, S.G., Kim H.C., Kwak, Y., Park, H.W., Kim, K.: Measurement of shoulder range of motion in patients with adhesive capsulitis. PLoS One 10(6) (2015)
22. Bo, A., Hayashibe, M., Poignet, P.: Joint angle estimation in rehabilitation with inertial sensors and its integration with Kinect. In: 33rd Annual International Conference of the IEEE Engineering in Medicine and Biology Society, EMBC 2011, pp. 3479–3483. IEEE Press, Boston (2011)
23. Fleiss, J.L.: The Design and Analysis of Clinical Experiments. Wiley Series in Probability and Mathematical statistics Applied Probability and Statistics, p. xiv-432. Wiley, New York (1986)

Author Index

Printed in the United States
By Bookmasters